The 21-Day High Fat Low Carb Diet Plan.

100+ Easy Low Carb Recipes

By Dan Barnett

Copyright © 2020 by Dan Barnett

All rights reserved.

No part of this book may be reproduced or transmitted in any form or by any means, electronic or mechanical, including photocopying, recording, or by any information storage and retrieval system, without permission in writing from the publisher.

Disclaimer

All material in "The 21-Day High Fat Low Carb Diet Plan. 100+ Easy Low Carb Recipes" is provided for your information only and may not be construed as medical advice or instruction. No action or inaction should be taken based solely on the contents of this information. Consult appropriate professionals for your health and well-being.

Remember that cooking is subjective. You may not achieve the results desired due to different brands of ingredients or different cooking abilities. Make sure you are not allergic to any ingredients.

CONTENTS

INTRODUCTION 8
- Low Carb Diet and Its Principles 8
- Low Carb vs Ketogenic Diet 9
- Who Is Suitable for HFLC Diet? 10
- Simple Rules for the High Fat Diet 11

WEEK 1 12
- Week 1 Shopping List 13

Day 1 14
- Cheddar Taco Crisps 15
- Greek Salad 16
- Avocado Chicken Roll 17
- Venison Spring Keto Stew 18
- Nuts' Keto Sweets and Peanut-Cream 19

Day 2 20
- Keto Cobb Salad 21
- Savory Bacon Cranberry Cheese Tartlets 22
- Marinated Olive with Cheese 23
- Burgundy Beef Stew 24
- Carrot Nut Cake 25

Day 3 27
- Fried Kale with Pork and Cranberries 28
- Buffalo Deviled Eggs 29
- Lemon and Blackberry Pudding 30
- Keto Pizza 31
- Roasted Turkey with Rosemary Thyme Gravy 33

Day 4 35
- Creamy Mashed Potatoes with Cauliflower 36
- Creamy Low Carb Butternut Squash Soup 37
- Pig Tongue 38
- Turkey Rolls and Vegetables 40
- Coconut Snowballs 42

Day 5 43

- Horseradish, Caramelized Onion and Cauliflower Mash ... 44
- Bacon and Eggs ... 45
- Celery Root with Mushrooms and Gorgonzola ... 46
- Keto Turkey Stew ... 47
- Nuts' Keto Sweets and Peanut-Cream ... 48

Day 6 ... 49
- Celery Crunch Salad ... 50
- Bok Choy Soup ... 51
- Dried Chicken Breast a la "Carpaccio" ... 52
- Stuffed Pork Tenderloin Wrapped in Bacon ... 53
- Coconut Snowballs ... 55

Day 7 ... 56
- Avocado and Chicken Salad with Bacon ... 57
- Cauliflower Cream Soup ... 58
- Buffalo Chicken Meatballs ... 59
- Beef Stew ... 60
- Vegan Chocolate Turron ... 62

WEEK 2 ... *63*
- Week 2 Shopping List ... 64

Day 8 ... 65
- Savory Bacon Cranberry Cheese Tartlets ... 66
- Broccoli Cheese Soup ... 68
- Avocado Chicken Roll ... 69
- Roasted Turkey with Rosemary Thyme Gravy ... 70
- "Ferrero Rocher" Keto Fat Bombs ... 72

Day 9 ... 73
- Spinach and Artichoke Casserole ... 74
- Keto Chicken Salad ... 75
- Buffalo Deviled Eggs ... 76
- Lamb Leg with Rosemary and Garlic ... 77
- Keto Pizza ... 78

Day 10 ... 80
- Avocado and Chicken Salad with Bacon ... 81
- Meat Soup ... 82

- Chocolate Fat Bombs with Sunflower Seeds 84
- Lamb Leg with Rosemary and Garlic 85
- Light Coconut Chocolate Bombs 86

Day 11 87
- Stuffed Mushrooms with Sausage 88
- Chorizo Soup 89
- Bacon and Cheese Cauliflower Muffins 90
- Creole Shrimp 91
- Georgian Pkhali 92

Day 12 93
- Stuffed Pork Tenderloin Wrapped in Bacon 94
- Chicken Curry Stew 96
- Cheddar Crisps 97
- Salmon and Asparagus with Onion-Mushroom Sauce 98
- Pumpkin Cheesecake Mousse 100

Day 13 101
- Walnuts Fennel and Goat Cheese Green Bean Salad 102
- Mushrooms with Chicken and Spices 103
- Buns with Oregano 104
- Green Chile Pork Stew 105
- Almond Cookies 107

Day 14 108
- Shrimp and Greens Salad 109
- French Onion Soup 110
- Pesto Mushrooms 112
- Beef Stew (low-carb) 113
- Lemon and Blackberry Pudding 114

WEEK 3 .... *115*
- Week 3 Shopping List 116

Day 15 117
- Keto Caesar Salad 118
- Keto Paleo Scotch Eggs 120
- Grilled Shrimp and Avocado 121
- Braised Beef and Zucchini 122

Vegan Chocolate Orange Truffles 123

Day 16 124
Keto Chicken Salad 125
Bacon Cheeseburger Soup 126
Coconut Oil Keto Bombs 128
Hearty Chicken Stew 129
Keto Chips with Zucchini 130

Day 17 131
Tuna, Greens, and Eggs Salad 132
Creamy Taco Soup (Low Carb) 133
Keto Easter "Cake" 135
Beef Stew 136
Festive Keto Terrine 138

Day 18 140
Tuna, Greens, and Eggs Salad 141
Wine-Coffee Beef Stew 142
Buffalo Deviled Eggs 143
Low Carb Pork Pie 144
Lemon Cheesecake 145

Day 19 146
Greek Salad 147
Creamy Chicken Bacon Soup (instant pot) 148
Raspberry Lemon Ice Bombs 149
Green Chile Pork Stew 150
Keto Livers Truffles 152

Day 20 153
Keto Cheese Rolls 154
Stroganoff High Fat Soup 155
Chocolate-Coconut Keto Candies 157
Venison Spring HFLC Stew 158
Chocolate Keto Ice Cream 159

Day 21 161
Stuffed Cheese Bell Pepper 162
Japanese Clear Onion Soup 163

Keto bombs with Philadelphia Cream Cheese 164
Low Carb Pork Pie 166
Chocolate Coconut Fat Bombs 167
Mass and Volume Conversion Rates 169

High Fat Low Carb Food List 170

INTRODUCTION

Low Carb Diet and Its Principles

The low-carb, high-fat eating plan, or LCHF diet, is promoted as a healthy and safe way to lose weight.

The Low Carb High Fat diet uses foods high in fat and proteins. In this case, carbohydrates (carbs) should be excluded entirely from the «keto» diet or reduced to a minimum in LCHF.

Originally, the Low Carb diet was developed for people with epilepsy and obesity. Now, it is actively used among athletes who want to tone their bodies to perfection. Women who dream of a more refined figure without having to do many physical exercises use the high fat low carb diet.

On a low carb diet, fat becomes the body's primary source of energy. This diet can include any fat, but carbohydrates should be reduced to zero. Carbohydrates enter the body and get processed into glucose, and glucose is very important for brain function and is the brain's primary fuel. Once there are no carbohydrates, and glucose, the body will start looking for an alternative source of fuel. This is fat, which is converted into fatty acids and ketone bodies.

Ketone bodies are a separate group of metabolic products. They are formed in the liver. Main types are acetone, acetoacetic acid, and beta-oxybutyric acid. In the keto diet and the HFLC diet, ketone bodies are the primary source of energy for the brain. When doing a keto diet, the body itself enters a special state: ketosis. In ketosis, the body is tuned to split fat to obtain ketone bodies constantly. So the person that is doing a high fat and low carbs diet actively consumes fat, but also actively loses it by feeding energy to the brain.

Low Carb vs Ketogenic Diet
What are the differences?

TYPE OF FOOD	LOW CARB	KETO
HIGH-FAT DAIRY (BUTTER, CREAM, CHEESE)	✓	✓
MILK/YOGURT	✓	MODERATION
FRUIT IN GENERAL	MODERATION	✗
LOW-SUGAR FRUIT (BERRIES, OLIVES, AVOCADO)	✓	MODERATION
FISH	✓	✓
MEAT	✓	✓
LEAFY GREEN VEGETABLES	✓	✓
NUTS	✓	MODERATION
ROOT VEGETABLES	✗	MODERATION
LEGUMES	MODERATION	✓
CANDY	✗	✗
DARK CHOCOLATE (IDEALLY 80% +)	✓	MODERATION
GRAINS, BREAD, AND GRAIN PRODUCTS	✗	✗
CRUCIFEROUS/GREEN VEGETABLES	✓	✗

The most notable difference between the ketogenic diet and LCHF diets is that the ketogenic diet has a strict limit on carbohydrates, while LCHF does not.

Who Is Suitable for HFLC Diet?

The ketogenic diet is effective for rapid weight loss when you need to lose extra pounds in a short period of time. Such a diet can easily control appetite and let you forget about being hungry for a long time.

This diet is not suitable for people:

- with gastrointestinal disease,
- any type of diabetes,
- liver and kidney disease,
- during pregnancy and lactation,
- when working in harsh and dangerous conditions,
- for people that do mentally demanding jobs.

In addition, athletes that want to gain muscle mass should not use it.

Before starting the ketogenic diet, it is absolutely necessary to consult with a doctor, as he/she will determine whether this diet suits you and your body.

High-Fat Diet Pros and Cons for Anyone Going Low-Carb

The most important advantage of a ketogenic diet is that it gives the ability to shed an impressive amount of excess weight in a very short time. For example, it is quite possible to lose 20 pounds in just 2 weeks! In this case, a person loses only fat, whereas muscle mass remains.

Simple Rules for the High Fat Diet

Our HFLC plan contains a lot of useful information that will help you begin the process of dieting. We made a menu for 21 days, and every one of 100 dishes have nutritional information.

For you to properly start the low carb diet and achieve results, you must follow the following recommendations:

- during the 1st week, the daily menu will have up to 40 grams of carbs per day to make it easier for you to start the diet; also in the 1st week you will be getting up to 40% of calories from carbohydrates;
- during the 2nd and 3d weeks, the daily menu will have up to 30 grams of carbs per day;
- during the low-calorie day avoid doing active sports.

Some useful keto friendly ideas:

- Get a lot of your calories from fat, a moderate amount from protein, and very few from carbs.
- Fat: 70% of calories/ Protein: 25% of calories/ Carbs: 5% of calories.
- Do not use «carbs» food, except for vegetables and avocados.
- Eat fatty meat.
- Add cheese, salad dressing, nuts, if you need to add a bit more into each meal to make sure you are reaching your goals.

WEEK 1

Week 1

MEAL	Breakfast	Lunch	Snacks	Dinner	Dessert
SUNDAY	Cheddar Taco Crisps	Greek Salad	Avocado Chicken Roll	Venison Spring Keto Stew	Nuts' Keto Sweets and Peanut-Cream
MONDAY	Keto Cobb Salad	Savory Bacon Cranberry Cheese Tartlets	Marinated Olive with Cheese	Burgundy Beef Stew	Carrot Nut Cake
TUESDAY	Fried Kale with Pork and Cranberries	Buffalo Deviled Eggs	Keto Pizza	Roasted Turkey with Rosemary Thyme Gravy	Lemon and Blackberry Pudding
WEDNESDAY	Creamy Mashed Potatoes with Cauliflower	Creamy Low Carb Butternut Squash Soup	Pig Tongue	Turkey Rolls and Vegetables	Coconut Snowballs
THURSDAY	Horseradish, Caramelized Onion and	Bacon and Eggs	Celery Root with Mushrooms and Gorgonzola	Keto Turkey Stew	Nuts' Keto Sweets and Peanut-Cream
FRIDAY	Celery Crunch Salad	Bok Choy Soup	Dried Chicken Breast a la "Carpaccio"	Stuffed Pork Tenderloin Wrapped in Bacon	Coconut Snowballs
SATURDAY	Avocado and Chicken Salad with Bacon	Cauliflower Cream Soup	Buffalo Chicken Meatballs	Beef Stew	Vegan Chocolate Turron

Week 1 Shopping List

PANTRY STAPLES
Butter
Butternut squash
Tuna – 8 cans
Campari tomatoes – 3 lb.
Almond flour - ½ lb.
Coconut flour – ½ cup
Coconut Milk – 2 pack

DAIRY & MEAT
Sour Cream – 1 container (16 oz.)
Soft Cream Cheese – 3 containers
Cheddar Cheese – 8 oz.
Eggs – 36 total
Bacon slices – 40 oz.
Blue Cheese – 1 cup
Chicken – 2 lb.
Chicken breast – 3 lb.
Gorgonzola cheese – 6 oz.
Ground pork – 1 lb.
Mozzarella – 16 oz.
Stew meat – 3 lb.
Turkey – 5 lb.
Pork tenderloin -1 lb.

Parmesan cheese – 3 oz.
Pig tongue – 4 lb.
Beef snack, tail – 5 lb.
Beef Stew – 2 lb.

VEGETABLES
Avocados – 2 total
Blackberries - ½ cup
Cranberries frozen – 12 oz.
Onions – 8 total
Celery - 1 package
Kale – 1 lb.
Lemon – 4 total
Cauliflower -2 lb.
Carrots – 7 total
Spinach – 2 oz.
Broccoli – 8 oz. frozen
Bok choy – 2 cup
Olives – 4 oz.

OTHER
Agave Syrup
Hazelnuts – 4 oz.
Mushrooms - 12 oz.
Pecans – 10 oz

Day 1

Cheddar Taco Crisps
Greek Salad
Avocado Chicken Roll
Venison Spring Keto Stew
Nuts Keto Sweets and Peanut-Cream

Fat - 101g   Carbs - 34g   Protein -84g   Calories -1364

Cheddar Taco Crisps
6 serves | 15 min

Ingredients

¾ cup full-fat Cheddar, finely shredded

¼ cup Parmesan, shredded

¼ tsp. chili powder

1/4 tsp. ground cumin

Large pinch of cayenne pepper

Directions

1. Preheat oven to 400 °F.
2. Line a baking sheet with a silicone-baking mat.
3. Mix the Cheddar, Parmesan, chili powder, cumin, and cayenne in a small bowl.
4. Place heaping tablespoonful's of the cheese mixture on the baking sheet 1 inch apart.
5. Spread out each pile, and pat down lightly.
6. Cook about 5 min. Bake until the cheese is golden brown and bubbly.
7. Let the crisps cool for a few seconds on the baking sheet.
8. Using a metal spatula, lift and drape the crisps over a rolling pin to cool completely.
9. Eat or store in an airtight container at room temperature for about 2 days.

Fat - 7g   Carbs - 1g   Protein -7g   Calories -88

Greek Salad

4 serves | 15 min

Ingredients

2 ripe tomatoes

½ cucumber

½ red onion

½ green bell pepper

7 oz. feta cheese

10 black olives

2 tbsp. olive oil

½ tbsp. red wine vinegar

2 tsp. dried oregano

Salt and pepper

Directions

Salad

1. Cut the tomatoes and cucumber into bite-sized pieces.
2. Thinly slice the bell pepper and onion.
3. Arrange the ingredients on a plate.
4. Add feta and olives.
5. Drizzle the salad with the dressing.
6. Sprinkle with oregano.

Dressing

Mix the olive oil and vinegar. Add salt and pepper to taste.

Fat - 20g   Carbs - 10g   Protein -9g   Calories -252

Avocado Chicken Roll
1 serves | 15 min

Ingredients

4 oz. fried chicken breast

1 tbsp. mayonnaise

½ medium avocado

salt

pepper

Directions

1. Cut the chicken into thin long strips.
2. Cut avocado into medium slices, put them in a plate, mix with mayonnaise and salt and pepper to taste.
3. Put avocado mixture on the meat strips. Roll strips.

Fat - 29g   Carbs - 13g   Protein -36g   Calories -450

Venison Spring Keto Stew
4 serves | 4 h 20 min

Ingredients

1 lb. venison	4 cups bone broth
2 tbsp. olive oil	1 tsp. salt
1 bulb garlic	1 tsp. pepper
1 cup shredded cabbage (purple)	2 cups chopped asparagus
1 cup sliced celery	2 bay leaves

Directions

1. At first, peel and slice garlic. Cut it into 1/8-inch thin slices.
2. Slice the purple cabbage.
3. Slice celery.
4. Preheat the skillet. Pour olive oil in it.
5. Add celery, garlic, bay leaves to the skillet. Saute the ingredients for about 5-6 minutes until tender.
6. Add venison to the cabbage. Salt and pepper. Cook until the meat is brown.
7. Take a big saucepan. Place cabbage, and venison in it, add broth.
8. Stew for 4 hours. Add water if the stew is dry.
9. When done, add chopped asparagus in the saucepan.
10. Serve the stew with olive oil and lime.

Fat - 16g   Carbs - 8g   Protein -32g   Calories -310

Nuts' Keto Sweets and Peanut-Cream

4 serves | 2 h 15 min

Ingredients

½ cup coconut oil

1 tbsp. cocoa powder

½ tsp. sweetener

Vanilla

Almonds, walnuts, peanuts, and/or hazelnuts

Peanut paste to taste

Butter to taste

Directions

1. Prepare a water bath. Melt coconut oil, but do not overheat.
2. Add cocoa and sweetener to melted oil. Add vanilla to taste. Stir. You can change the number of ingredients if you want. Pour half the contents into molds.
3. Put the nut or peanut-cream filling in each candy. Cover with rest of coconut oil mixture and sprinkle cocoa powder on the sweets with nuts immediately. Place in the refrigerator to harden.
4. Wait for the bottom layer of the candy to cool before stuffing. Mix ¼ lb. of paste and 1 oz. of oil (or your choice). Add to the thickened bottom layer of chocolates. Then cover with the second part of the mixture.
5. Put the candy in the fridge. Keep the keto-candies in the cold.

Fat - 29g   Carbs – 2.4g   Protein -1g   Calories -264

Day 2

Keto Cobb Salad
Savory Bacon Cranberry Cheese Tartlets
Marinated Olive with Cheese
Burgundy Beef Stew
Carrot Nut Cake

Fat – 144 g   Carbs - 37g   Protein -75g   Calories -1543

Keto Cobb Salad
4 serves | 20 min

Ingredients

2 cherry tomatoes

½ avocado

1 hard-boiled egg

2 cups mixed green salad

2 oz. cooked chicken breast

1 oz. feta cheese

¼ cup cooked bacon

1 tbsp. olive oil

½ tbsp. white wine vinegar

Salt and pepper

Directions

1. Cut the tomatoes, egg, and avocadoes into slices.
2. Shred cooked chicken breast.
3. Crumble feta cheese.
4. Place the mixed green salad into salad bowl or on a plate.
5. Place tomatoes, avocado, egg, bacon, cheese, and chicken on top of the salad.

Dress the salad with olive oil and white wine vinegar. Salt and pepper to taste. You can use one tbsp Ranch dressing.

Fat - 15g   Carbs – 7g   Protein -10g   Calories -190

Savory Bacon Cranberry Cheese Tartlets

6 serves | 1 h

Ingredients

Tart crust

1 cup blanched almond flour

1 egg

1/5 cup butter melted

1/8 tsp. sea salt

Filling

3 chopped bacon slices

1/2 cup cubed Mahon Menorca Semi-Cured cheese

2 oz. unsweetened dried cranberries

1 tsp. fresh thyme leaves

Salt

Black pepper to taste

Directions

1. Preheat oven to 370°F. Grease 6-cup muffin pan.
2. Combine the ingredients for the crust. Form dough.
3. Make 6 balls with your hands. Place one into each cup.
4. Press dough with a small glass to make the tart crusts.
5. Bake the crusts for 7 minutes until lightly golden. Remove them from the oven.
6. Fill the crusts with fried and chopped bacon, cubed Mahon Menorca cheese, and dried cranberries.
7. Sprinkle the tartlets with salt, pepper, and fresh thyme leaves.
8. Bake for 10 minutes or until cheese is completely melted.
9. Remove the tartlets and cool for 10 minutes.

Fat - 26g   Carbs – 8g   Protein -19g   Calories -158

Marinated Olive with Cheese
8 serves | 8 h 30 min

Ingredients

4 oz. cream cheese, cold

5 oz. sharp white Cheddar cheese

1 ½ oz. pimiento-stuffed olives

1 ½ oz. pitted Greek olives

1 oz. cup balsamic vinegar

1 oz. olive oil

1 tsp. fresh parsley, minced

1 tsp. fresh basil, minced

1 garlic cloves, minced

1 oz. canned pimiento strips, drained and chopped

Directions

1. Cut the cheese in half lengthwise. Cut each half into 1/4-inch slices.
2. Arrange cheeses upright in a ring on a serving plate. Alternate cheddar and cream cheese slices.
3. Place olives in the center of the plate.
4. Whisk vinegar, oil, parsley, basil, and garlic in a small bowl until blended.
5. Drizzle the seasoning over olives and cheese.
6. Sprinkle the ingredients with the pimientos.
7. Cool at least 8 hours or overnight in the refrigerator.

Fat - 16g   Carbs – 2g   Protein -6g   Calories -168

Burgundy Beef Stew
6 serves | 2 h 10 min

Ingredients

2 tbsp. avocado oil	¼ medium onion
2 lb. beef stew chunks	2 tbsp. cumin powder
2 bacon slices	1 tbsp. turmeric
4 cup bone broth	1 tbsp. garlic powder
2 small carrots	1 tsp. ginger powder
4 oz. green beans	Salt and pepper to taste

Directions

1. Peel and chop the carrots, onion, beans.
2. Chop beef chunks into small pieces.
3. Dice bacon slices.
4. Take a large pot and pour olive oil in it. Brown the beef stew chunks in the oil over high heat.
5. Add vegetables, spices to the beef. Cover the pot; simmer the stew on medium heat for 90 min. Stir occasionally.
6. Season stew with salt and pepper.
7. Meanwhile, take a small skillet. Preheat it. Fry bacon until crispy, for 2-3 minutes.
8. Add frying bacon to the ready stew.

Fat - 41g   Carbs – 3g   Protein -27g   Calories -507

Carrot Nut Cake
4 serves | 1 h 10 min

Ingredients

2 oz. almond flour

1 oz. coconut flour

2 tbsp. baking powder

2 oz. pecan

2 tbsp. chia seeds

4 oz. grated carrot

4 chicken eggs

3 oz. Philadelphia cream cheese

3 oz. sour cream (30%)

3 oz. butter

Vanilla, cinnamon, salt

Directions

1. Preheat oven to 320°F.
2. Prepare the cream. In a blender, place the cream cheese, sour cream and vanilla to taste. Mix everything well until smooth. Allow the mixture to sit.
3. Mix almond and coconut flour, chia seeds and pecans. Add baking powder, salt, and cinnamon. Grind all these dry ingredients in the flour. You can leave large pieces.
4. Grated carrot.

5. Separate the yolks in the eggs. Beat the eggs white to add air. Mix the yolks.
6. Melt the butter and let cool. Mix the egg whites with the yolks. Add creamy melted butter. Mix again.
7. In the mixture add dry Ingredients mix flour, nuts and seeds. Gently stir manually or with a blender.
8. Fold the carrots evenly into the batter.
9. Place the batter onto a baking sheet and bake in the oven for 45 min.
10. Cool the cake and cut into several layers. Smear each layer with cream. Let the cake rest overnight in the refrigerator.

Fat - 46g   Carbs – 17g   Protein -13g   Calories -520

Day 3

Fried Kale with Pork and Cranberries

Buffalo Deviled Eggs

Keto Pizza

Roasted Turkey with Rosemary Thyme Gravy

Lemon and Blackberry Pudding

Fat - 113g   Carbs - 40g   Protein -150g   Calories -1848

Fried Kale with Pork and Cranberries
4 serves | 20 min

Ingredients

3 oz. butter

1 lb. kale

2/3 lb. smoked pork belly or bacon

2 oz. walnuts or pecans

½ cup frozen cranberries

Salt and black pepper to taste

Directions

1. Rinse, trim, and chop kale into large chunks. Set aside.
2. Use the strips of bacon or cut the pork into strips. Fry over medium heat until golden brown and crispy.
3. Place kale into the pan. Fry 3-5 minutes until wilted.
4. Add salt and pepper to taste. Turn off the heat.

Add cranberries and nuts to the kale and bacon or pork. Stir the ingredients.

Fat - 56g   Carbs – 17g   Protein -34g   Calories -692

Buffalo Deviled Eggs
6 serves | 20 min

Ingredients

6 hard boiled chicken eggs, large

½ lb. boiled and chopped chicken

¼ onion

2 oz. blue cheese crumbles

2 oz. Franks Buffalo Wing Sauce

1 small chopped celery

2 tbsp. blue cheese dressing

Directions

1. Boil the eggs.
2. Chop the chicken and celery.
3. Peel cooked and cooled eggs. Cut them in half lengthwise. Separate the yolks from the egg whites and place yolks in mixing bowl.
4. Add chicken, celery, blue cheese, Franks Buffalo Wing Sauce and dressing to yolks.
5. Press the onion and add juice to the bowl. Mix all the ingredients.
6. Stuff the egg whites with yolk mixture using a fork or spoon.
You can also pipe the yolks into the whites using a Ziploc bag with the tip cut off.

Fat - 18g   Carbs – 2g   Protein -19g   Calories -253

Lemon and Blackberry Pudding

4 serves | 35 min

Ingredients

2 oz. coconut flour

5 chicken eggs

2 tbsp. butter

2 tbsp. coconut oil

2 tbsp. oily cream

2 tbsp. erythritol

1 lemon

2 tsp. lemon juice

1/2 cup blackberries

1/4 tsp. baking powder

10 drops liquid stevia

Directions

1. Preheat oven to 345 °F.
2. Separate egg yolks from whites. Whisk the yolks to a pale yellow color. Add erythritol and stevia and mix until evenly combined.
3. Add fatty cream, coconut oil, and lemon juice.
4. Wash and zest the lemon. Add zest to the mixture and mix.
5. Add the coconut flour and baking powder. Mix all the ingredients.
6. Add the blackberry to the mixture. Press the berries into it a little.
7. Bake pudding for 20-25 min. in the baking cups.

Fat - 14g   Carbs – 16g   Protein -6g   Calories -177

Keto Pizza
8 serves | 1 h

Ingredients

Sauce

1/3 cup canned sugar-free crushed tomatoes

1 tsp. olive oil

1 small clove garlic, minced

A pinch of kosher salt

Keto Dough

1 ½ cups shredded Mozzarella

2 tbsp. full-fat sour cream

2/3 cup almond flour

2 large eggs, lightly beaten

A pinch of kosher salt

Olive oil

Toppings

1/3 cup shredded whole-milk Mozzarella

Crushed red pepper flakes and dried oregano, for sprinkling

Directions

Sauce

1. Combine the tomatoes, minced garlic, and salt in a small bowl.
2. Let the mixture sit for 30 min. at room temperature.

Dough

1. Place the cheese and sour cream in a large microwave-safe bowl.
2. Microwave the ingredients in one-minute intervals, stirring until the cheese is melted. Cool the mixture slightly.
3. Add the eggs, flour, and ¼ tsp. of salt to the cheese mixture. Mix with your hands until a stretchy, slightly wet dough forms.

Pizza

1. Adjust an oven rack to the low position and place a baking sheet on it.
2. Preheat oven to 450 °F.
3. Grease a piece of parchment paper with olive oil.
4. Lightly coat your hands in oil and place the dough on the parchment, patting into a ¼-inch-thick rectangle. Make the edges a bit thicker to create a crust all around.
5. Place the dough on the baking sheet. Bake until puffy and golden. Cook about 15 min.
6. Remove the dough from the oven and top with sauce and mozzarella. Bake pizza until it's heated through and cheese is melted, about 5 min.
7. Remove the dough from the oven.
8. Sprinkle with pepper flakes, salt, and oregano.

Fat - 5g   Carbs – 1g   Protein -4g   Calories -160

Roasted Turkey with Rosemary Thyme Gravy
6 serves | 4 h 30 min

Ingredients

<u>Roasted Turkey</u>

4 lb. whole turkey

½ small onion

1 small lemon

¼ cup minced garlic

1 tsp. dried rosemary

2 chopped stalks green onions

<u>Turkey Coating</u>

2 tbsp. melted butter

1 tsp. cayenne

1 tsp. chicken herb seasoning

<u>Gravy</u>

Leftover parts of turkey

1/5 cup chicken stock

1.5 cups water

1 tsp. Worcestershire

1 stalks green onions

2 Brussels sprouts

1 tbsp. bacon fat

2 sprigs fresh thyme

1 bay leaf

¼ tsp. xanthan gum

2 oz. heavy cream

Salt and pepper

Directions

1. Preheat oven to 325 °F. Stuff the turkey with onion, lemon, minced garlic, dried rosemary, and chopped green onions.
2. Mix the coating ingredients. Brush the turkey with this mixture.
3. Bake turkey for 150 minutes.
4. Boil the turkey innards in water and chicken broth for 1 hour.
5. Add brussels sprouts. Green onion, Worcestershire, salt, and pepper to the gravy. Boil for 30-45 minutes. Then blend gravy.
6. Add sprigs of fresh thyme, bay leaf, and heavy cream. Bring to a rolling boil.
7. Stir Continuously. Let gravy reduce for 15-20 minutes. It should be relatively thick. Add the xanthan gum, and mix well. Let turkey rest. Serve with gravy.

Fat - 20g   Carbs – 3g   Protein -88g   Calories -566

Day 4

Creamy Mashed Potatoes with Cauliflower
Creamy Low Carb Butternut Squash Soup
Pig Tongue
Turkey Rolls and Vegetables
Coconut Snowballs
Fat - 120g   Carbs - 43g   Protein -95g   Calories -1680

Creamy Mashed Potatoes with Cauliflower
3 serves | 30 min

Ingredients

2/3 lb. riced cauliflower

½ cup sour cream

3 tbsp. heavy whipping cream

3 tbsp. butter

¼ tbsp garlic powder

4 tbsp. Parmesan cheese

2 tbsp. chopped chives

Salt and pepper

Directions

1. Place the cauliflower on a deep plate, and cover with paper towel. Microwave cauliflower for 5 minutes. You can roast or steam it too. Cauliflower must be slightly soft.
2. Add sour cream, heavy whipping cream, butter, garlic powder, Parmesan cheese, salt, pepper to taste. Mix the ingredients with an immersion blender.
3. Add 1 tbsp. of chopped chives to the mixture. Mix well.
4. You can serve the dish with mashed potatoes and 1 tbsp. chives.

Fat - 28g   Carbs – 8g   Protein -7g   Calories -300

Creamy Low Carb Butternut Squash Soup
8 serves | 1 h 10 min

Ingredients

2 lb. butternut squash, cut in half without seeds

2 tbsp. avocado oil

Sea salt

Black pepper

2 minced cloves of garlic

2 tbsp. fresh thyme

½ tsp. cinnamon

1/8 tsp. nutmeg

4 cups chicken bone broth (or broth to your taste)

13.5-oz. can coconut milk (370g)

Directions

1. Preheat the oven to 400 °F. Line a baking sheet with parchment paper. Place the butternut squash halves open side up on the baking sheet.
2. Drizzle butternut squash with 1 tbsp. of avocado oil. Sprinkle with sea salt and black pepper. Flip over, face down.
3. Roast it in the oven for 40-55 minutes.
4. Take a large pot. Heat 1 tbsp. of avocado oil in it over medium heat.
5. Add minced garlic, nutmeg, thyme, cinnamon. Saute for 1 minute.
6. Add the broth, coconut milk. Cook for 20 minutes.
7. Scoop the squash. Add it into the soup. Puree until smooth with the immersion blender.
8. Saute on the low heat for 3 minutes. Serve.

Fat - 12g   Carbs – 4g   Protein -4g   Calories -183

Pig Tongue
6 serves | 50 min

Ingredients

2 lb. pig tongue

1 stick cinnamon

2 pieces badian

5 peppercorns black pepper

2 bay leaves

1 pinch of chili pepper

1 clove garlic

1 oz. celery root

3-4 pinches of salt

For cranberry sauce

½ lb. cranberries, fresh or frozen

2 tsp. sugar

1 pinch of salt

2 tsp. water

Directions

1. Wash the pork tongue and place in a saucepan. Cover with water, add the spices, and bring to a boil.
2. Boil on a medium heat for 35-40 min.
3. Remove from the heat. Rinse the tongue with cold water and peel.
4. Place the cranberries in saucepan. Add sugar, salt, and water.
5. Cook the ingredients on medium heat for 15 min.
6. Sieve the cranberry mass. If the sauce is too thin, reduce over low heat.
7. Cut pork tongue into thin slices; serve on a plate with cranberry sauce on top.

Fat - 47g   Carbs – 7g   Protein -61g   Calories -712

Turkey Rolls and Vegetables
4 serves | 30 min

Ingredients

1 lb. turkey breast

½ lb. cream cheese

1 avocado

1 bell pepper

1 cucumber

1 tbsp. mayonnaise

1 garlic clove

Lemon juice

Salt

Pepper

Directions

1. Wash and dry the turkey breast, if necessary.
2. Mix the lemon juice, chopped garlic, and pepper. Place the turkey on a deep plate. Pour lemon juice over it and leave for two hours.
3. From time to time turn the turkey to soaking well.
4. Preheat the oven to 350°F.
5. Place the turkey on a baking sheet. Bake for 30-40 minutes in the oven.
6. Cool the turkey.

7. Put slightly softened cream cheese into a plate. Stir with a mixer to a creamy consistency.
8. Peel the avocado. Mush with a fork, and add a couple drops of lemon juice and salt.
9. Mix avocado and cream cheese. Add a spoonful of mayo. Stir again with a mixer. You should get a thick sauce.

    Cut pepper and cucumber into thin strips.
10. Slice baked and cooled turkey. Spread cheese and avocado sauce on the turkey with.
11. Put pieces of pepper and cucumber on meat. Make small rolls.

Fat - 30g   Carbs – 16g   Protein -23g   Calories -420

Coconut Snowballs
5 serves | 10 min

Ingredients

2 oz. shredded coconut

1 oz. almond flour

1 ½ oz. agave syrup

Directions

1. Mix 1 ½ oz. shredded coconut, flour, and syrup in a food processor until well combined.
2. Make 10 balls using your hands.
3. Roll the balls in ½ oz. shredded coconut.

You can keep these balls in a sealed container in a fridge for one week.

Fat - 4g   Carbs – 8g   Protein -1g   Calories -65

Day 5

Horseradish, Caramelized Onion and Cauliflower Mash

Bacon and Eggs

Celery Root with Mushrooms and Gorgonzola

Keto Turkey Stew

Nuts' Keto Sweets and Peanut-Cream

Fat - 110g   Carbs - 31g   Protein -40g   Calories -1221

Horseradish, Caramelized Onion and Cauliflower Mash

8 serves | 50 min

Ingredients

1 medium onion

1 large cleaned, trimmed cauliflower

2 tbsp. minced garlic

2 tbsp. olive oil

2 tbsp. butter

¼ cup sour cream

¼ cup creamy horseradish

Salt (sea) and pepper to taste

Directions

1. In a large sauté pan, place onions, garlic, olive oil, butter, salt and pepper. Cook over medium-low heat until onion caramelizes, about 30 minutes.
2. While onion caramelizes, add 4 cups water to a large sauce pan. Steam the cauliflower for 15 minutes over high heat. Then, drain the water and remove in the sauce pan.
3. Mash the cauliflower in the pan with the fork. Add caramelized onion, horseradish sauce, and sour cream to the pan. Mix all the ingredients well.

Fat - 10g   Carbs – 4g   Protein -1g   Calories -147

Bacon and Eggs
10 serves | 15 min

Ingredients

5 eggs

3 tbsp. Homemade Mayonnaise

2 slices bacon (thick cut)

1 tbsp. pickle relish (sugar free)

Directions

1. Peel hard-boiled eggs. Cut each in half lengthwise. Fry bacon.
2. Separate the yolks from the egg whites. Crumble yolks with a fork in a large bowl.
3. Then add Mayonnaise to the yolks. Mix until the mixture looks like batter.
4. Add pickle relish. Mix all the ingredients again.
5. Cool and crumble bacon. Add it to the yolk mixture.
6. Fill the eggs' halves with the yolk. Use fork for this.
7. You can sprinkle the deviled eggs with paprika.

Fat - 5g   Carbs – 2g   Protein -4g   Calories -67

Celery Root with Mushrooms and Gorgonzola
4 serves | 50 min

Ingredients

1 lb. celery root	3 tbsp. butter
3 tbsp. olive oil	1 red onion, chopped
¼ lb. mushrooms	1/3 oz. Gorgonzola cheese
3 oz. spinach leaves	Salt and pepper, to taste
3 oz. hazelnut	

Directions

1. Preheat oven to 400 °F.
2. Wash and peel the celery root. Cut the root into slices or rings, 1 to 1 1/2 cm thick.
3. Smear both sides of slices with olive oil, salt, and pepper
4. Place parchment paper on the baking sheet. Put the celery on the parchment and bake in the oven for 40-45 min. until the celery becomes soft and golden.
5. Fry the mushrooms in butter until brown. Add salt and pepper.
6. Place the hazelnuts in a dry pan and fry for 5-7 min. Then, cool and chop nuts in half.
7. To make salad, mix spinach leaves, chopped red onion, mushrooms and hazelnuts in a bowl.
8. Put the salad on the cooked celery. Top with a piece of cheese and a drizzle of olive oil.

Fat - 42g   Carbs – 19g   Protein -14g   Calories -428

Keto Turkey Stew
5 serves | 5 h

Ingredients

1 lb. of turkey thighs and leg meat, diced

1 clove garlic, crushed

1 tbsp. olive oil

2 oz. bacon, diced

½ tsp. salt

½ tsp. white ground pepper

1/3 lb. button mushrooms

1/2 cup heavy cream

1 leek, halved and sliced

1 tbsp. fresh thyme leaves

1/2 tsp. xanthan gum

1 tbsp. whole grain mustard

¼ cup parsley, roughly chopped

Directions

1. Brown the turkey meat in the olive oil in a large non-stick frying pan over high heat. Then shift it into a slow cooker.
2. Fry garlic, leek and bacon for 3-5 minutes until the leek has softened.
3. Add this mixture to the meat along with thyme, salt, pepper, and mushrooms.
4. Mix the xanthan gum, mustard, and cream. Then send it to the slow cooker, while stirring well.
5. Cook for 2 hours on high heat.
6. Stir through the parsley and serve alone or with a side of Creamy Broccoli Mash.

Fat - 24g   Carbs – 4g   Protein -20g   Calories -315

Nuts' Keto Sweets and Peanut-Cream

4 serves | 15 min

Ingredients

½ cup coconut oil

1 tbsp. cocoa powder

½ tsp. sweetener

vanilla

almonds, walnuts, peanuts, and/or hazelnuts

peanut paste to taste

butter to taste

Directions

1. Prepare a water bath. Melt coconut oil, but do not overheat.
2. Add cocoa and sweetener to melted oil. Add vanilla to taste. Stir. You can change the number of ingredients if you want. Pour half the contents into molds.
3. Put the nut or peanut-cream filling in each candy. Cover with rest of coconut oil mixture and sprinkle cocoa powder on the sweets with nuts immediately. Place in the refrigerator to harden.
4. Wait for the bottom layer of the candy to cool before stuffing. Mix 100 g of paste and 30 g of oil (or your choice). Add to the thickened bottom layer of chocolates. Then cover with the second part of the mixture.
5. Put the candy in the fridge. Keep the keto-candies in the cold.

Fat - 29g   Carbs – 3g   Protein -1g   Calories -264

Day 6

Celery Crunch Salad

Bok Choy Soup

Dried Chicken Breast a la "Carpaccio"

Stuffed Pork Tenderloin Wrapped in Bacon

Coconut Snowballs
Fat - 83g   Carbs - 40g   Protein -126g   Calories -1411

Celery Crunch Salad
```
4 serves | 10 min
```

Ingredients

8 stalks celery (with leaves)	1 chopped green onion
1 green apple	¼ cup extra virgin olive oil
2 oz. crumbled blue cheese	1 tbsp. Dijon mustard
1 cup chopped pecans	½ lemon (juice)
2 oz. parsley	2 tbsp. white wine vinegar

Directions

Salad

1. Wash and chop celery into medium slices. Place slices in a large bowl.
2. Wash and cut apple into thin slices. Add slices to the bowl.
3. Chop parsley and add to the bowl.
4. Chop pecans. Add the pecans to the bowl.
5. Add blue cheese, green onion to the mixture.
6. Drizzle the dressing over the top of the salad.

Dressing

1. In separate bowl, mix mustard, lemon juice, and vinegar.
2. Whisk the ingredients and drizzle with olive oil. Add salt and pepper.

Fat - 28g   Carbs – 13g   Protein -5g   Calories -303

Bok Choy Soup
1 serves | 5 min

Ingredients

2 bok choy stalks

1 cup vegetable broth

1 tsp. nutritional yeast

2 pinch garlic powder

2 pinch onion powder

Salt and pepper to taste

Directions

1. Take a bowl. Mix all ingredients in it.
2. Place the bowl in a microwave for 3 minutes.

Fat - 2g   Carbs – 7g   Protein -9g   Calories -73

Dried Chicken Breast a la "Carpaccio"

4 serves | 6 h 10 min

Ingredients

2 1/3 lb. chicken breast

5 tsp. salt

2 tsp. coriander

1/2 tsp. spices, to taste

1 tsp. black pepper

3 tsp. sweet pepper

Paprika

Directions

1. Cut each half of a chilled breast lengthwise into two parts. You'll have 4 long thick pieces.
2. Pat each piece dry with a paper towel.
3. Mix the spices and crush before drying chicken.
4. Roll each chicken piece in spices until well coated and salt lightly.
5. Put the chicken in a container, pressing the pieces down.
6. Place the container in the refrigerator for 6-8 hours.
7. After cooling cut a small piece of rinse and taste. Taste a small piece of chicken to see if it is too salty. If it's not too salty, rinse the chicken under water. If it is salty, soak the chicken for 30 min. before rinsing. Then, rinse again and dry.
8. Cut the chicken into pieces, cover pieces in paprika. Then, string pieces on skewers for kebabs. Hang these skewers to dry at room temperature for 12-16 hours.

Fat - 7g   Carbs – 8g   Protein -54g   Calories -315

Stuffed Pork Tenderloin Wrapped in Bacon

4 serves | 1 h

Ingredients

1 lb. pork tenderloin

14 slices bacon

2 tsp. minced garlic

½ small onion (50-100 g)

2 oz. spinach

3 oz. cream cheese

1 tbsp. olive oil

¾ tsp. liquid smoke

¾ tsp. dried thyme and rosemary

salt and pepper

For Vegetable Sauté

4 oz. chopped broccoli

½ orange bell pepper

½ cup diced tomatoes

½ tsp. onion and garlic powder

salt and pepper

Directions

1. In a frying pan, cook onion in olive oil until soft (a few minutes).
2. Add garlic. Chop for 60 seconds. Then, add spinach, ¼ tsp. dried thyme and rosemary and salt and pepper to taste.
3. Preheat oven to 355 °F.
4. Lay pork tenderloin on the cutting board. Pound it with meat hammer until flat. Shape tenderloin into a square and season with salt and pepper. Add liquid smoke.
5. Make a bacon weave the same size as the tenderloin.
6. Spread cream cheese and spinach on the pork tenderloin. Place these ingredients on top of bacon. Roll up.
7. Season stuffed pork with salt, pepper, ¼ tsp. of thyme and rosemary.
8. Hold together the bacon ends with toothpicks if it's necessary. Place roll in the frying pan.
9. Bake it for 75-90 minutes.
10. For garnish stew broccoli, peppers, and tomatoes in the fat in the bottom of the pan after baking pork.

Fat - 43g   Carbs – 4g   Protein -57g   Calories -655

Coconut Snowballs
5 serves | 10 min

Ingredients

2 oz. shredded coconut

1 oz. almond flour

1 ½ oz. agave syrup

Directions

1. Mix 1 ½ oz. shredded coconut, flour, and syrup in a food processor until well combined.
2. Make 10 balls using your hands.
3. Roll the balls in ½ oz. shredded coconut.

You can keep these balls in a sealed container in a fridge for one week.

Fat - 4g   Carbs – 8g   Protein -1g   Calories -65

Day 7

Avocado and Chicken Salad with Bacon
Cauliflower Cream Soup
Buffalo Chicken Meatballs
Beef Stew
Vegan Chocolate Turron
Fat - 136g   Carbs - 40g   Protein -127g   Calories -1388

Avocado and Chicken Salad with Bacon
4 serves | 15 min

Ingredients

1 slice bacon

½ medium avocado

¼ lb. chicken breast

1 oz. cheddar cheese

1 hard-boiled egg

½ lb. Romaine lettuce

1 tbsp. olive oil

1 tbsp. apple cider vinegar

Salt and pepper

Directions

1. Chop the lettuce. Place into salad bowl.
2. Chop bacon, avocado, chicken breast, Cheddar cheese, and egg. Place the ingredients atop the lettuce.
3. Add oil and vinegar. Sprinkle salt and pepper.

Fat - 13g   Carbs – 4g   Protein -9g   Calories -189

Cauliflower Cream Soup

2 serves | 35 min

Ingredients:

½ lb. cauliflower

2 oz. onions

1 oz. butter

1 oz. cheese

1/3 lb. chicken broth

1 oz. fatty cream

Salt and pepper to taste

Directions:

1. Peel and cut onion well.
2. On the frying pan cook the onion until it is golden brown.
3. In a big pot, boil the cauliflower and, cook for 15 minutes.
4. Blend cooked cauliflower in the food processor.
5. Add chicken broth, fried onions, cream, chopped cauliflower in the saucepan. Add grated cheese. Boil for 10 minutes.
6. Add salt and spices to taste.

Fat - 19g   Carbs – 9g   Protein -9g   Calories -229

Buffalo Chicken Meatballs

4 serves | 30 min

Ingredients

1 lb. organic chicken

1 egg, beaten

2 green onions, chopped

1 celery stalk, chopped finely

1 tbsp. almond flour or coconut flour

1 tbsp. organic mayonnaise

1 tsp. onion powder

1 tsp. garlic powder

1 tsp. natural salt

1 tsp. pepper

1 cup Buffalo sauce for wings

Directions

1. Preheat oven to 400 °F. Grease a baking sheet with coconut oil (or butter or avocado oil).
2. In a large bowl, mix all ingredients, except the buffalo sauce.
3. Make 2-inch balls from the mixture. Place the meatballs on the baking sheet. Bake for 15 min.
4. Remove the meatballs from the oven.
5. Place the meatballs in the skillet over the medium heat.
6. Add the buffalo sauce to the skillet. Cook until the sauce is warmed through.

Fat - 75g   Carbs – 8g   Protein -40g   Calories -333

Beef Stew
6 serves | 4 h

Ingredients

5 lb. beef snack, tail

3 medium carrots

8 Campari tomatoes

2 medium onions

1 tsp. tomato sauce

8 cloves garlic

2 tsp. garlic powder

2 tbsp. apple cider vinegar

4 cups chicken broth

2 cups water

2 tsp. onion powder

4 tsp. salt

3 tsp. crushed red pepper

2 tsp. parsley

1 tsp. cayenne

2 tsp. black pepper

2 tsp. basil

3 whole bay leaves, spices, to taste

Directions

1. Pell and cut carrots, tomatoes, onion, garlic into chunky pieces.
2. Preheat the frying pan over medium heat.
3. Place vegetables and spices on the frying pan, stir and cook until translucent.
4. Replace the ingredients in the soup pot.
5. Take another cast iron skillet. Place beef snack in it . Cook on both sides, until crispy.
6. Pour broth into the pot to the onion, carrot and garlic.
7. Add two cups of water, apple cider vinegar. Cook for 2-3 minutes. Stir.
8. Add tomatoes, tomato sauce. Stir well.
9. Submerge beef tails into the broth. Boil the ingredients.
10. Reduce the heat to a simmer. Cover the pot.
11. Slightly simmer on a low heat for 3 hours.
12. When meat is cooked, it will be very soft and tender.
13. Remove the bay leaves from the pot. Serve.

Fat - 22g   Carbs – 9g   Protein -68g   Calories -531

Vegan Chocolate Turron
8 serves | 15 min +chill time

Ingredients

1/3 lb. dark chopped chocolate

1 tbsp. melted coconut oil

1 oz. unsalted raw hazelnuts

Directions

1. Place dark chocolate in a saucepan. Cook over medium heat, stirring occasionally until chocolate is melted.
2. Remove chocolate from the heat. Add hazelnuts, and combine well.
3. Pour the chocolate-hazelnuts mixture into lined rectangular dish.
4. Cool to room temperature. Chop the turron.
5. If it's too hot in the room, keep turron in the fridge.

Fat - 8g   Carbs – 10g   Protein -1g   Calories -106

WEEK 2

Week 2

MEAL	Breakfast	Lunch	Snacks	Dinner	Dessert
SUNDAY	Savory Bacon Cranberry Cheese Tartlets	Broccoli Cheese Soup	Avocado Chicken Roll	Roasted Turkey with Rosemary Thyme Gravy	"Ferrero Rocher" Keto Fat Bombs
MONDAY	Spinach and Artichoke Casserole	Keto Chicken Salad	Buffalo Deviled Eggs	Lamb Leg with Rosemary and Garlic	Keto Pizza
TUESDAY	Avocado and Chicken Salad with Bacon	Meat Soup	Chocolate Fat Bombs with Sunflower Seeds	Lamb Leg with Rosemary and Garlic	Light Coconut Chocolate Bombs
WEDNESDAY	Stuffed Mushrooms with Sausage	Chorizo Soup	Bacon and Cheese Cauliflower Muffins	Creole Shrimp	Georgian Pkhali
THURSDAY	Stuffed Pork Tenderloin Wrapped in Bacon	Chicken Curry Stew	Cheddar Crisps	Salmon and Asparagus with Onion-Mushroom Sauce	Pumpkin Cheesecake Mousse
FRIDAY	Walnuts Fennel and Goat Cheese Green Bean Salad	Mushrooms with Chicken and Spices	Buns with Oregano	Green Chile Pork Stew	Almond Cookies
SATURDAY	Shrimp and Greens Salad	French Onion Soup	Pesto Mushrooms	Beef Stew (low-carb)	Lemon and Blackberry Pudding

Week 2 Shopping List

PANTRY STAPLES
Butter
Almond flour - 1 lb.
Coconut flour – 1/3 cup
Coconut Milk – 2 pack

DAIRY & MEAT
Heavy Cream – 10 oz.
Soft Cream Cheese – 4 containers (24 oz.)
Goat cheese – 8 oz.
Cheddar Cheese – 20 oz.
Eggs – 23 total
Bacon slices – 54 oz.
Pork tenderloin – 1 lb.
Italian sausage – 8 oz.
Chicken – 3 lb.
Chicken breast – 24 oz.
Mozzarella – 16 oz.
Leg of bone – in lag – 8 lb.
Turkey – 3 lb.
Ground pork - 2 lb.
Parmesan cheese – 9 oz.
Diced tomatoes – 3 lb.

Beef Stew – 1 lb.

VEGETABLES
Avocados – 3 total
Artichoke hearts – 1 lb.
Brussels sprouts – 2 total
Green beans – 1 lb.
Onions – 13 total
Lemon – 3 total
Cauliflower - 2 lb.
Carrots – 2 total
Spinach – 11 oz.
Broccoli – 32 oz. frozen
Olives – 8 oz.

OTHER
Hazelnuts – 12 oz.
Mushrooms – 30 oz.
Salmon - 1 lb.
Shrimp – 1 lb.
Walnuts – 8 oz.
Champignons -12 oz.

Day 8

Savory Bacon Cranberry Cheese Tartlets
Broccoli Cheese Soup
Avocado Chicken Roll
Roasted Turkey with Rosemary Thyme Gravy
"Ferrero Rocher" Keto Fat Bombs
Fat - 116g   Carbs -29g   Protein -152g   Calories -1772

Savory Bacon Cranberry Cheese Tartlets
6 serves | 30 min

Ingredients

<u>Tart crust</u>

1 cups blanched almond flour

1 egg

1/5 cup butter melted

Sea salt

<u>Filling</u>

3 chopped bacon slices

½ cups cubed Mahon Menorca Semi-Cured Cheese

1/4 cup unsweetened dried cranberries

1 tsp. fresh thyme leaves

Salt

Black pepper to taste

Directions

1. Preheat oven to 370°F. Grease 6-cup muffin pan.
2. Combine the ingredients for the crust. Form dough.
3. Make 6 balls with your hands. Place one into each cup.
4. Press dough with a small glass to make the tart crusts.
5. Bake the crusts for 7 minutes until lightly golden. Remove them from the oven.
6. Fill the crusts with fried and chopped bacon, cubed Mahon Menorca cheese, and dried cranberries.
7. Sprinkle the tartlets with salt, pepper, and fresh thyme leaves.
8. Bake for 10 minutes or until cheese is completely melted.
9. Remove the tartlets and cool for 10 minutes.

Fat - 33g   Carbs – 7g   Protein -11g   Calories -360

Broccoli Cheese Soup
8 serves | 20 min

Ingredients

4 cups broccoli

4 cloves of minced garlic

3 ½ cups vegetable broth

1 cup heavy cream

3 cups shredded cheddar cheese

Directions

1. Saute garlic for 1 minute in a large pot over medium heat. Cook until fragrant.
2. Add chicken broth, chopped broccoli, heavy cream. Increase heat to a boil. After that reduce heat, simmer for 20 minutes until broccoli are tender.
3. Add shredded cheddar cheese gradually. Stir constantly until melted. Make very low heat to simmer. Remove the pot from the heat immediately once all the cheese is melted.

Fat - 20g   Carbs – 5g Protein -15g Calories -257

Avocado Chicken Roll

1 serves | 15 min

Ingredients

¼ lb. fried chicken breast

1 tbsp. mayonnaise

½ medium avocado

Salt

Pepper

Directions

1. Cut the chicken into thin long strips.
2. Cut avocado into medium slices, put them in a plate, mix with mayonnaise and salt and pepper to taste.
3. Put avocado mixture on the meat strips. Roll strips.

Fat - 30g   Carbs – 13g   Protein -36g   Calories -449

Roasted Turkey with Rosemary Thyme Gravy
6 serves | 4 h 30 min

Ingredients

<u>Roasted Turkey</u>

Whole turkey 4 lb.

½ small onion

1 small lemon

1/8 cup minced garlic

1 tsp. dried rosemary

2 chopped stalks green onions

<u>Turkey Coating</u>

2 tbsp. melted butter

1/2 tsp. cayenne

1 tsp. chicken herb seasoning

<u>Gravy</u>

Leftover parts of turkey

1 ½ oz. chicken stock

1 ½ cups water

1 tsp. Worcestershire

1 stalks green onions

2 Brussels sprouts

1 tbsp. bacon fat

2 sprigs fresh thyme

1 bay leaf

1/8 tsp. xanthan gum

1/8 cup heavy cream

Salt and pepper

Directions

1. Preheat oven to 325 °F. Stuff the turkey with onion, lemon, minced garlic, dried rosemary, and chopped green onions.
2. Mix the coating ingredients. Brush the turkey with this mixture.
3. Bake turkey for 150 minutes.
4. Boil the turkey innards in water and chicken broth for 1 hour.
5. Add brussels sprouts. Green onion, Worcestershire, salt, and pepper to the gravy. Boil for 30-45 minutes. Then blend gravy.
6. Add sprigs of fresh thyme, bay leaf, and heavy cream. Bring to a rolling boil.
7. Stir Continuously. Let gravy reduce for 15-20 minutes. It should be relatively thick. Add the xanthan gum, and mix well.
8. Let turkey rest. Serve with gravy.

Fat - 20g   Carbs – 3g   Protein -88g   Calories -566

"Ferrero Rocher" Keto Fat Bombs
7 serves | 1 h 15 min

Ingredients

1 1/2 oz. ground hazelnuts

1 oz. coconut oil

Erythritol powder

1 1/2 oz. sugar-free chocolate

1/2 tsp. sugar-free vanilla extract

1 tsp. cocoa powder

Chopped hazelnuts and 7 whole hazelnuts

Directions

1. Melt the sugar-free chocolate in a double boiler.
2. Melt the coconut oil in the microwave if needed.
3. Add the chopped hazelnuts, powdered erythritol, melted coconut oil, cocoa powder, and vanilla extract into a food processor and blend on high for approximately 30–45 seconds.
4. Add the melted chocolate and blend for another 15 seconds.
5. Cool down the mixture in the freezer, then form 7 small balls with your hands.
6. Push a whole hazelnut into the middle of each fat bomb and roll the balls in chopped hazelnuts. Refrigerate.

Fat - 14g   Carbs – 1g   Protein -2g   Calories -140

Day 9

Spinach and Artichoke Casserole
Keto Chicken Salad
Buffalo Deviled Eggs
Lamb Leg with Rosemary and Garlic
Keto Pizza
Fat - 138g   Carbs -27g   Protein -151g   Calories -1972

Spinach and Artichoke Casserole
8 serves | 50 min

Ingredients

½ lb. cream cheese

¼ cup homemade mayonnaise

1/3 lb. shredded Parmesan cheese

1 tbsp. minced garlic

1 tsp. crushed basil

1 lb. artichoke hearts

½ lb. spinach

½ lb. mozzarella cheese

Salt and paper to taste

Directions

1. Preheat oven to 350°F
2. Melt cream cheese in the microwave.
3. Add the mayo to the melted cream cheese. Combine the ingredients.
4. Add shredded Parmesan, garlic, and basil. Mix the ingredients. Add salt and pepper.
5. Chop the artichoke and add it to the other ingredients. Mix well.
6. Cut the spinach and combine with the artichoke mixture.
7. Grease a baking sheet with oil. Placed the mixture on baking sheet.
8. Cover the top of the dish with shredded mozzarella. Bake the casserole for 30 minutes.

Fat - 17g   Carbs – 10g   Protein -12g   Calories -233

Keto Chicken Salad
1 serves | 20 min

Ingredients

2/3 lb. chicken breast

3 oz. thin-cut bacon slices

½ lb. avocado

½ oz. mixed leaf greens

4 tsp. Paleo Ranch Dressing

Duck fat for greasing

Directions

1. Preheat the oven to 400°F.
2. Crisp the chicken breasts. Season with salt and pepper.
3. Grease pan with fat. Place breasts skin side down on the pan. Fry for 5-6 minutes. Flip the chicken and cook 30 seconds. Than transfer pan in the oven. Cook 10-15 minutes, until chicken is cooked through.
4. Place the slices bacon on the bake sheet. Bake the bacon slices in the oven until crispy. Alternatively, crisp the bacon in a frying pan.
5. Remove chicken from the oven. Cool for 5 minutes.
6. Slice the avocado and cooked chicken.
7. Place leafy greens on the plate. Add avocado, crispy bacon and sliced chicken.
8. Top with Ranch dressing.

Fat - 48g   Carbs – 12g   Protein -48g   Calories -627

Buffalo Deviled Eggs

6 serves | 20 min

Ingredients

6 hard boiled chicken eggs, large

1/3 lb. boiled and chopped chicken

¼ onion

2 oz. blue cheese crumbles

2 oz. Franks Buffalo Wing Sauce

1 small chopped celery

2 tbsp. blue cheese dressing

Directions

1. Boil the eggs.
2. Chop the chicken and celery.
3. Peel cooked and cooled eggs. Cut them in half lengthwise. Separate the yolks from the egg whites and place yolks in mixing bowl.
4. Add chicken, celery, blue cheese, Franks Buffalo Wing Sauce and dressing to yolks.
5. Press the onion and add juice to the bowl. Mix all the ingredients.
6. Stuff the egg whites with yolk mixture using a fork or spoon. You can also pipe the yolks into the whites using a Ziploc bag with the tip cut off.

Fat - 12g   Carbs – 2g   Protein -29g   Calories -152

Lamb Leg with Rosemary and Garlic
6 serves | 2 h 30 min

Ingredients

4 lb. leg of bone-in lamb

1 sliced cloves garlic

1 thinly sliced lemons

3 fresh rosemary sprigs

Salt and pepper

1 tsp. oil

Directions

1. Preheat the oven to 350°F. Grease the baking sheet.
2. With a knife, make 1/2-inch-deep slits all over the lamb (about 25 cuts).
3. Stuff the garlic into the slits.
4. Mix 1 tsp. salt and ½ tsp. pepper. Season lamb with this mixture. Leave meat at room temperature for 45 minutes.
5. Place the slices lemon on the sheet so they overlap. They will keep the meat from burning. Place one rosemary sprigs on the lemon and lamb. Place 2 sprigs on the top of the lamb.
6. Bake lamb for 1 ½ to 2 hours. Baste with the pan juice every 15 minutes.
7. Loosely tent the lamb with the foil. Let rest. Slice perpendicular to the bone

Fat - 56g   Carbs – 2g   Protein -58g   Calories -800

Keto Pizza
8 serves | 1 h

Ingredients

Sauce

1/3 cup canned sugar-free crushed tomatoes

1 tsp. olive oil

1 small clove garlic, minced

A pinch of kosher salt

Keto Dough

1 ½ cups shredded Mozzarella

2 tbsp. full-fat sour cream

2/3 cup almond flour

2 large eggs, lightly beaten

A pinch of kosher salt

Olive oil

Toppings

1/3 cup shredded whole-milk Mozzarella

Crushed red pepper flakes and dried oregano, for sprinkling

Directions

<u>Sauce</u>

1. Combine the tomatoes, minced garlic, and salt in a small bowl.
2. Let the mixture sit for 30 min. at room temperature.

<u>Dough</u>

1. Place the cheese and sour cream in a large microwave-safe bowl.
2. Microwave the ingredients in one-minute intervals, stirring until the cheese is melted. Cool the mixture slightly.
3. Add the eggs, flour, and ¼ tsp. of salt to the cheese mixture. Mix with your hands until a stretchy, slightly wet dough forms.

<u>Pizza</u>

1. Adjust an oven rack to the low position and place a baking sheet on it.
2. Preheat oven to 450 °F.
3. Grease a piece of parchment paper with olive oil.
4. Lightly coat your hands in oil and place the dough on the parchment, patting into a ¼-inch-thick rectangle. Make the edges a bit thicker to create a crust all around.
5. Place the dough on the baking sheet. Bake until puffy and golden. Cook about 15 min.
6. Remove the dough from the oven and top with sauce and mozzarella. Bake pizza until it's heated through and cheese is melted, about 5 min.
7. Remove the dough from the oven.
8. Sprinkle with pepper flakes, salt, and oregano.

Fat - 5g   Carbs – 1g   Protein -4g   Calories -160

Day 10

Avocado and Chicken Salad with Bacon

Meat Soup

Chocolate Fat Bombs with Sunflower Seeds

Lamb Leg with Rosemary and Garlic

Light Coconut Chocolate Bombs

Fat – 279   Carbs -25   Protein – 97   Calories - 2166

Avocado and Chicken Salad with Bacon

4 serves | 20 min

Ingredients

1 slice bacon

½ medium avocado

¼ lb. chicken breast

1 oz. cheddar cheese

1 hard-boiled egg

½ lb. Romaine lettuce

1 tbsp. olive oil

1 tbsp. apple cider vinegar

Salt and pepper

Directions

1. Chop the lettuce. Place into salad bowl.
2. Chop bacon, avocado, chicken breast, Cheddar cheese, and egg. Place the ingredients atop the lettuce.
3. Add oil and vinegar. Sprinkle salt and pepper.

Fat - 13g   Carbs – 4g   Protein -9g   Calories -189

Meat Soup

6 serves | 50 min

Ingredients

8 slices bacon

4 cups fried broccoli

½ large sliced onion

2 cups shredded cheddar cheese

2 cups chicken broth

¼ cup shredded Parmesan

2 tbsp. butter

2 tbsp. coconut flour

½ cup heavy cream

2 tsp. minced garlic

½ tsp. salt

1 tsp. cayenne pepper

Directions

1. Fry bacon over medium heat for 5-7 minutes in a frying pan.
2. Chop the onion.
3. Remove the bacon on a paper towel. Leave 3 tbsp. of bacon fat in the pan.
4. Add butter, onion, and garlic to the pan, and fry for 4-5 minutes until onion is translucent.
5. Add coconut flour to the pan and cook for 1 minute.
6. Mix cream and milk in a bowl. Add the mixture to the pan and wait until it starts to bubble. Mix well and reduce heat to medium level.
7. Add cheddar cheese and parmesan to the pan, and mix well. Cook for 2-3 minutes on low heat, then add broccoli and cook for 2-3 minutes.
8. Add bacon and cook for 5 minutes. Turn off the heat.
9. Mix the ingredients in the pan with the blender, then add broth, cayenne pepper and mix again.
10. Turn on medium heat. Simmer the soup for 20-30 minutes, stirring it every 5 minutes.

Fat - 40g   Carbs – 8g   Protein -20g   Calories -476

Chocolate Fat Bombs with Sunflower Seeds

4 serves | 40 min

Ingredients

3 ½ oz. of sunflower seeds, roasted and ground

7 oz. butter, melted

2 tsp. sweetener (for example, Stevie)

3 tbsp. cocoa powder

Vanilla or vanilla extract to taste

Directions

1. Mix all dry ingredients.
2. Add melted butter and vanilla, and stir well.
3. Pour the mixture into silicone molds and refrigerate.

Note: It is essentially a bombshell. There are 91.7% fat, 4% protein, 4.2% carbohydrate.

Fat - 24g   Carbs – 3g   Protein -3g   Calories -232

Lamb Leg with Rosemary and Garlic
6 serves | 2 h 30 min

Ingredients

4 lb. leg of bone-in lamb

1 sliced cloves garlic

1 thinly sliced lemons

3 fresh rosemary sprigs

Salt and pepper

1 tsp. oil

Cooking

1. Preheat the oven to 350°F. Grease the baking sheet.
2. With a knife, make 1/2-inch-deep slits all over the lamb (about 25 cuts).
3. Stuff the garlic into the slits.
4. Mix 1 tsp. salt and ½ tsp. pepper. Season lamb with this mixture. Leave meat at room temperature for 45 minutes.
5. Place the slices lemon on the sheet so they overlap. They will keep the meat from burning. Place one rosemary sprigs on the lemon and lamb. Place 2 sprigs on the top of the lamb.
6. Bake lamb for 1 ½ to 2 hours. Baste with the pan juice every 15 minutes.
7. Loosely tent the lamb with the foil. Let rest. Slice perpendicular to the bone

Fat - 56g   Carbs – 2g   Protein -58g   Calories -800

Light Coconut Chocolate Bombs
10 serves | 10 min

Ingredients

1 cup of macadamia nuts, salted

1–2 tbsp. coconut oil (melted, for most solid fat bombs)

½ tsp. vanilla extract (optional)

1/6 cup powdered sweetener

1/8 cup cocoa powder

Directions

1. Put the macadamia nuts in a food processor or high-power blender and pulse them into small pieces.
2. Add melted coconut oil and vanilla, if using, to the nuts. Mash until a butter is formed.
3. Pour the cocoa powder and sweetener onto the paste gradually while stirring. Mix the ingredients until smooth.
4. Place pieces of parchment paper into mini-cupcake molds. Spoon the dough evenly into the molds.
5. Freeze for about 30 minutes to harden.

Note: use salted macadamia nuts. If you have unsalted, add sea salt to taste.

Fat - 45g   Carbs – 9g   Protein -8g   Calories -469

Day 11

Low calories day. Try to limit physical activity today.

Stuffed Mushrooms with Sausage
Chorizo Soup
Bacon and Cheese Cauliflower Muffins
Creole Shrimp
Georgian Pkhali
Fat -123 g   Carbs -34 g   Protein -63g   Calories -1138

Stuffed Mushrooms with Sausage
6 serves | 45 min

Ingredients

10-12 large mushrooms

½ lb. Italian sausage, sliced

1 small onion

1/3 lb. grated Parmesan cheese

2 oz. cup Italian bread crumbs

½ tsp. minced garlic

1/2 tsp. chopped fresh parsley

Directions

1. Preheat oven to 350°F.
2. Hollow out mushroom caps, save scrapings.
3. Heat frying pan over medium-high heat. Add sausage, onion, and reserved mushroom scrapings. Cook and stir the ingredients 4-6 minutes until sausage is browned.
4. Drain and discard liquid. And fry again.
5. Add 4 oz. g Parmesan cheese, bread crumbs, garlic, and parsley to sausage mixture. Cook 3-5 minutes.
6. Cool sausage mixture. Stuff each mushroom cap with mixture. Place the stuffed caps on a baking sheet. Bake for 12 minutes. Then sprinkle remaining 2 oz. Parmesan cheese over mushrooms. Bake until cheese is melted and bubbling, about 3 minutes.

Fat - 10g   Carbs – 3g   Protein -11g   Calories -142

Chorizo Soup
6 serves | 1 h 10 min

Ingredients

1 tsp. extra virgin olive oil

2 onions, finely chopped

2 cloves of garlic, minced

1 green bell pepper, finely chopped

3 oz. chorizo

3 cups jarred or fresh tomatoes, finely diced

2 cups chicken broth

½ red pepper flakes

1 tsp. fresh cilantro to taste

¾ cup cheddar cheese to taste

Organic tortilla to taste

Directions

1. Chop onions, garlic, tomatoes, and pepper with a knife. Or use a food processor until finely chopped.
2. Take a stock pot, place it over medium-high heat.
3. Cut and crumble the chorizo.
4. Place garlic, bell pepper, chorizo, onions in the pot.
5. Saute soup's ingredients until onion is brown.
6. Stir tomatoes, broth, pepper flakes in the stock pot.

Fat - 12g   Carbs – 10g   Protein -10g   Calories -202

Bacon and Cheese Cauliflower Muffins
6 serves | 45 min

Ingredients

1/3 lb. chopped cauliflower

2 oz. grated Cheddar cheese

1 large chicken eggs

4 pieces bacon

½ oz. almond flour

½ oz. feta cheese

1/4 tsp. baking powder

1 tsp. garlic powder

1 tsp. celery

1 tsp. oregano

1 tsp. paprika

Salt and pepper, to taste

Directions

1. Preheat oven to 400 °F.
2. Grind the cauliflower and place in a large bowl. Add the dry ingredients, bacon, and cheese.
3. Add eggs, mix thoroughly until mixture forms.
4. Place the mixture in cupcake molds.
5. Sprinkle with feta cheese.
6. Bake for 35 min.

Fat - 8g   Carbs – 3g   Protein -8g   Calories -115

Creole Shrimp
4 serves | 30 min

Ingredients

½ lb. large shrimp

½ lb. smoked sausage, (can be replaced with shrimp)

1/4 cup olive or canola oil

1/4 cup celery, diced

1 medium onion, chopped

1 small bell pepper, chopped

2 tsp. garlic, minced

1-2 tsp. fresh thyme+

2 tsp. creole seasoning or more

½ -1 lb. stew tomatoes or 2-3 fresh tomatoes

2 cups or more broth/water

1 tsp. Worcestershire sauce

1 tsp. bouillon powder, optional+1 bay leaf

1-2 green onions, chopped

2 tbsp. parsley, chopped

Directions

1. Sauté shrimp with creole seasoning and 1 tbsp. oil over medium heat in a heavy bottomed dutch for about 1-2 minutes.
2. Add sausage and saute until browned on both sides. Remove aside.
3. Fry onions, celery, green pepper, thyme and garlic with remaining oil, while stiring for about 2-3 minutes.
4. Top up leaf creole spice, tomatoes, chicken broth, and Worcestershire sauce. Simmer for 10-15 minutes. Add bouillon as needed.
5. Pout out shrimp with sausage to the dutch, mix all ingredients and cook for about 2-3 minutes.
6. Serve with white rice or fettuccine garnishing parsley.

Fat - 68g   Carbs – 9g   Protein -21g   Calories -391

Georgian Pkhali

3 serves | 2 h 15 min

Ingredients

1 cup walnuts

1 bunch spinach, roughly chopped

1 bunch parsley, roughly chopped

2 cloves garlic, peeled

½ tsp. salt

Lemon juice to taste

Directions

1. Soak the nuts in water for at least 2 hours.
2. Drain and rinse the nuts, then blend in a food processor.
3. Peel the garlic.
4. Cut the greens.
5. Add garlic and greens. Blend until a homogeneous mixture forms.
6. Add lemon juice and salt to taste.
7. Roll into medium balls.

Fat - 25g   Carbs – 9g   Protein -14g   Calories -288

Day 12

Stuffed Pork Tenderloin Wrapped in Bacon
Chicken Curry Stew
Cheddar Crisps
Salmon and Asparagus with Onion-Mushroom Sauce
Pumpkin Cheesecake Mousse
Fat -162 g   Carbs - 25g   Protein -121g   Calories -2072

Stuffed Pork Tenderloin Wrapped in Bacon
4 serves | 1 h

Ingredients

1 lb. pork tenderloin

14 slices bacon

2 tsp. minced garlic

½ small onion

2 oz. spinach

3 oz. cream cheese

1 tbsp. olive oil

¾ tsp. liquid smoke

¾ tsp. dried thyme and rosemary

Salt and pepper

For Vegetable Sauté

1/3 lb. chopped broccoli

½ orange bell pepper

½ cup decide tomatoes

½ tsp. onion and garlic powder

Salt and pepper

Directions

1. In a frying pan, cook onion in olive oil until soft (a few minutes).
2. Add garlic. Chop for 60 seconds. Then, add spinach, ¼ tsp. dried thyme and rosemary and salt and pepper to taste.
3. Preheat oven to 355°F.
4. Lay pork tenderloin on the cutting board. Pound it with meat hammer until flat. Shape tenderloin into a square and season with salt and pepper. Add liquid smoke.
5. Make a bacon weave the same size as the tenderloin.
6. Spread cream cheese and spinach on the pork tenderloin. Place these ingredients on top of bacon. Roll up.
7. Season stuffed pork with salt, pepper, ¼ tsp. of thyme and rosemary.
8. Hold together the bacon ends with toothpicks if it is necessary. Place roll in the frying pan.
9. Bake it for 75-90 minutes.
10. For garnish stew broccoli, peppers, and tomatoes in the fat in the bottom of the pan after baking pork.

Fat - 43g   Carbs – 4g   Protein -57g   Calories -655

Chicken Curry Stew
4 serves | 40 min

Ingredients

1 ½ lb. boneless chicken thighs

2 tbsp. curry powder

2 tsp. garlic powder

1/3 cup coconut oil

1 lb. cauliflower

1 green bell pepper

2 cups coconut milk

Salt and pepper

¼ cup fresh cilantro/parsley

Directions

1. Cut chicken thighs into medium pieces.
2. Cut cauliflower, peppers into small pieces.
3. Heat coconut oil in the big frying pan or a wok.
4. Add curry and garlic powder. Fry for 1-2 minutes.
5. Add chicken to the skillet, add salt and pepper.
6. Sauté the ingredients for 5 minutes, while stirring often. Cook until golden brown and cooked through.
7. Remove from the pan, keep chicken warm.
8. Place cauliflower, bell pepper in the skillet. Fry vegetables on medium high heat for 3-5 minutes.
9. Add coconut milk to the vegetables, cook for 5-10 minutes.
10. Add salt, pepper, fried chicken to the pan and cook for 1 minute.
11. Use chopped cilantro for serving.

Fat - 68g   Carbs – 9g   Protein -33g   Calories -781

Cheddar Crisps
4 serves | 15 min

Ingredients

4 tbsp. shredded Cheddar cheese

Directions

1. Preheat oven to 350°F.
2. Line bake sheet with parchment paper.
3. Drop the shredded cheese on paper. Make sure that there are 2 inches between the drops of the cheese.
4. Bake 10-15 minutes until the edges of the crisps brown.
5. Turn off the oven, remove the sheet. Cool the crisps for 10-15 minutes.

Fat - 2g   Carbs – 0g   Protein -2g   Calories -28

Salmon and Asparagus with Onion-Mushroom Sauce

4 serves | 40 min

Ingredients

1 lb. salmon

¼ lb. champignons

1 onion

1 garlic clove

2 tbsp. olive oil

½ cup sesame oil

Salt

Basil

Pepper

Directions

<u>Marinade</u>

Mix sesame oil with finely chopped garlic, basil, pepper, and salt.

Salmon and Asparagus

1. Cut the salmon, and put into a small saucepan. Pour the marinade over fish and chill in the refrigerator for an hour.
2. Preheat the oven to 355 °F. Cover a baking sheet with foil.
3. Put the slices of salmon and washed asparagus on the baking sheet. Cover them with foil.
4. Bake fish and vegetables in the oven for 15-20 minutes.
5. Wash, peel, and cut champignons. Mince the onion. Fry the ingredients in olive oil until browned.
6. Remove the fish and asparagus from the oven, and top with mushroom and onion mixture. Bake for another 10 minutes.

Fat - 42g   Carbs – 3g   Protein -25g   Calories -478

Pumpkin Cheesecake Mousse

6 serves | 10 min + chill time

Ingredients

1/3 lb. softened cream cheese

½ lb. unsweetened pumpkin puree

1/3 cup erythritol

1 tsp. pure vanilla extract

1 tbsp. pumpkin pie spice

1/2 cup heavy cream

Directions

1. In a large mixing bowl, combine the cream cheese and pumpkin puree by hand. The mixture must be creamy, smooth, and without clumps.
2. Add vanilla, spices, erythritol, and heavy cream to the pumpkin mixture. Combine well.
3. The mousse must set in the refrigerator before it can be served.

Fat - 8g   Carbs – 9g   Protein -4g   Calories -130

Day 13

Walnuts Fennel and Goat Cheese Green Bean Salad
Mushrooms with Chicken and Spices
Buns with Oregano
Green Chile Pork Stew
Almond Cookies
Fat - 73g   Carbs - 35g   Protein -75g   Calories -1210

Walnuts Fennel and Goat Cheese Green Bean Salad

6 serves | 40 min

Ingredients

1 tbsp. Dijon mustard

1 tbsp. white wine vinegar

1/2 tsp. kosher salt

¼ tsp. freshly ground black pepper

2 oz. extra-virgin olive oil

1 lb. trimmed green beans

1 small fennel bulb

1/2 cup walnuts

½ lb. fresh Goat cheese

Directions

Salad

1. Boil salted water in a large saucepan. Add the green beans. Cook for 6-8 minutes.
2. Drain and cool under cold water.
3. Slice the fennel bulb into half-moons.
4. Toast and coarsely chop walnuts.
5. Crumble the goat cheese.
6. Combine the green beans, fennel, and walnuts. Before serving add the goat cheese.
7. Top with dressing.

Dressing

Whisk mustard, salt, vinegar, and pepper. Add the oil and combine.

Fat – 27g   Carbs – 11g   Protein -17g   Calories -228

Mushrooms with Chicken and Spices

4 serves | 2 h

Ingredients

2/3 lb. ceps	Thyme
½ lb. raw chicken meat	Basil
1 cup chicken broth	Oregano
1 tbsp. butter	Salt
2 tbsp. fatty whipped cream	Pepper
1 clove of garlic	

Directions

1. Wash and peel ceps well. Separate the caps from the legs.
2. Preheat the frying pan. Add mushrooms and fry for 5 minutes over low heat.
3. Cut chicken into large chunks. Add them to the mushrooms.
4. Add the broth. Season the ingredients with finely chopped garlic, a pinch of basil, thyme, oregano, pepper and salt.
5. Simmer for about 1.5 hours on low heat. Then, add butter and whipped cream.

Fat – 7g   Carbs – 7g   Protein -19g   Calories -173

Buns with Oregano
6 serves | 30 min

Ingredients

4 eggs

4 tbsp. olive oil

2 oz. almond flour

¼ tsp. salt

1 tbsp. dried oregano

Directions

1. Preheat oven to 390°F.
2. Thoroughly mix the eggs, olive oil, flour, ¾ of the oregano, and the salt.
3. Pour the mixture into a 6-cup muffin mold.
4. Sprinkle with the remaining oregano.
5. Bake for 25 min. Then, cool at room temperature before removing the buns from molds.

Fat – 11g   Carbs – 1g   Protein -7g   Calories -131

Green Chile Pork Stew
8 serves | 1 h 45 min

Ingredients

2 lb. pork loin

2 tsp. ground cumin

2 tsp. granulated garlic

1 tsp. pure ground chile powder (to taste)

2 oz. chopped onion

2 cloves garlic

1 ½ lb. can whole hatch green chilies and liquid

3 tbsp. oil

2 cups water

poached eggs optional

salt to taste

Directions

1. Cut pork loin into cubes.
2. Preheat oil in a big frying pan. Fry pork until brown.
3. Add spices to the pork. Cook until fragrant.
4. At the same time, chop garlic and onion. Place ingredients in a food processor.
5. Add canned chilies to the food processor. Mix and make thick chunky paste.

6. Add chili and onion mixture to the pork. Pour the liquid of canned chilies.

7. Pour two cups of water.

8. Stir the ingredients and make low-heat. Cover the pan with a lid.

9. Simmer the stew for 60-90 minutes until pork is tender.

10. Add a little water during the last hour cooking.

11. Before finishing, add salt to taste.

12. Serve stew with the poached eggs.

Fat – 10g   Carbs – 4g   Protein -20g   Calories -182

Almond Cookies
4 serves | 45 min

Ingredients

2 cups almond flour

1/2 cup erythritol

2 oz. butter

2 chicken eggs

1 tsp. extract of vanilla

1 tsp. cinnamon

Salt and halves of almonds

Directions

1. Preheat the oven to 355 °F.
2. While the oven is heating, mix almond flour, erythritol, cinnamon, and a pinch of salt in a bowl.
3. Beat the eggs in a small bowl. Add butter and vanilla. Stir.
4. Mix the dry ingredients with the egg mixture until evenly combined.
5. Form dough into small circles using a spoon.
6. Decorate circles with half an almond.
7. Line a baking sheet with parchment paper coated in butter. Put the cookies on it.

Bake for 10-15 minutes.

Fat – 18g   Carbs – 12g   Protein -12g   Calories -496

Day 14

Shrimp and Greens Salad
French Onion Soup
Pesto Mushrooms
Beef Stew (low-carb)
Lemon and Blackberry Pudding
Fat - 121g   Carbs - 24g   Protein -63g   Calories -1414

Shrimp and Greens Salad
4 serves | 20 min

Ingredients

½ lb. peeled frozen shrimp

2 oz. salad

1 oz. olives

2 tbsp. butter

2 tbsp. olive oil

1 garlic clove

Lemon juice

Salt

Pepper

Directions

1. Thaw the shrimp at room temperature or rinse with hot water. If you chose the second method, then use a colander. Rinse shrimp carefully.
2. Transfer the shrimps to a deep plate, add finely chopped garlic, lemon juice, salt and pepper. Mix well. Marinate the shrimp for 5-10 minutes.
3. Pre-heat a pan and add butter. Squeeze the shrimp a little. Lay shrimp in the frying pan. Fry the shrimp for 8-10 minutes.
4. Cool the shrimp.
5. Roughly chop the lettuce leaves. Put chopped leaves onto a large plate.
6. Add the shrimp and olives.
7. Season the ingredients with olive oil. Add salt and pepper to taste.

Fat – 14g   Carbs – 1g   Protein -9g   Calories -158

French Onion Soup
8 serves | 1 h

Ingredients

¾ cup expeller-pressed coconut oil (or butter)

3-4 large sweet onions, sliced

6-10 minced cloves of fresh garlic

2 tbsp. arrowroot powder

½ cup red wine

2-3 tsp. dried thyme

5 large bay leaves

1 ¼ tsp. sea salt

½ tsp. black pepper

½ tsp. garlic powder

½ tsp. onion powder

½ tsp. garlic powder

½ tsp. onion powder

6 cups organic beef stock

Directions

1. In a large saucepan place the coconut oil. Add thinly sliced onion, garlic. Cover the saucepan and stir occasionally. Cook for about 10 minutes over medium heat until onions are translucent.

2. Add arrowroot powder for coating the onions.

3. Add red wine, stirring around. Cook for 3-4 minutes to burn off the alcohol.
4. Add spices and stir.
5. Add beef stock and cook for 5-7 minutes.
6. Reduce the heat to medium-low, simmer for 45 minutes.
7. Remove from heat. Serve.
8. Top the soup with cheese (Parmesan or Swiss) to taste.

Fat – 14g   Carbs – 1g   Protein -9g   Calories -158

Pesto Mushrooms
5 serves | 45 min

Ingredients

½ lb. champignon

2/3 lb. bacon

3 oz. cream cheese, softened

1 oz. pesto with basil

Directions

1. Preheat oven to 350 °F.
2. In a bowl, mix the cream cheese with the pesto sauce.
3. Place the bacon strips on a cutting board and cut strips in half lengthwise.
4. Peel the mushrooms and remove the stems.
5. Fill each mushroom cap with the cream cheese mixture and pesto.
6. Wrap a narrow strip of bacon around each mushroom. Wind the second strip around each cap in the other direction, so the mushroom is covered with bacon.
7. Place the mushrooms on the baking sheet and put in preheated oven.
8. Bake for 20-30 min. until the bacon is crispy and a pleasant golden brown.

Fat – 33g   Carbs – 3g   Protein -25g   Calories -409

Beef Stew (low-carb)
4 serves | 1 h 10 min

Ingredients

- 1 lb. beef short rib
- 4 cloves garlic
- 2 cups beef broth
- ¼ lb. carrot
- 1/4 tsp. pink Himalayan salt
- ¼ lb. onion
- ¼ lb. radishes
- 1/2 tsp. xanthan gum
- 1/4 tsp. pepper
- 1 tbsp. butter
- 1 tbsp. coconut oil

Directions

1. Put chopped ribs along with salt and pepper on the heated large saucepan with coconut oil and brown them from all sides. Once cooked, set aside.
2. Boil chopped onions along with garlic and butter. Mix it with broth when onions are tender.
3. Add xanthan gum and combine.
4. Put meat in the boiling broth and cook for 30 minutes with the lid closed.
5. After that time, add chopped carrots and radishes and boil for another 30 minutes. Stir it during that time.
6. Once the broth has thickened, the dish is ready. You can add water or bullion, if it is very thick.
7. Stew should be served warm.

Fat – 37g   Carbs – 6g   Protein -19g   Calories -432

Lemon and Blackberry Pudding

6 serves | 1 h 10 min

Ingredients

2 oz. coconut flour

5 chicken eggs

2 tbsp. butter

2 tbsp. coconut oil

2 tbsp. oily cream

2 tbsp. erythritol

1 lemon

2 tsp. lemon juice

1/2 cup blackberries

1/4 tsp. baking powder

10 drops liquid stevia

Directions

1. Preheat oven to 345 °F.
2. Separate egg yolks from whites. Whisk the yolks to a pale yellow color. Add erythritol and stevia and mix until evenly combined.
3. Add fatty cream, coconut oil, and lemon juice.
4. Wash and zest the lemon. Add zest to the mixture and mix.
5. Add the coconut flour and baking powder. Mix all the ingredients.
6. Add the blackberry to the mixture. Press the berries into it a little. Bake pudding for 20-25 minutes.

Fat – 18g   Carbs – 4g   Protein -7g   Calories -158

WEEK 3

MEAL	Breakfast	Lunch	Snacks	Dinner	Dessert
SUNDAY	Keto Caesar Salad	Keto Paleo Scotch Eggs	Grilled Shrimp and Avocado	Braised Beef and Zucchini	Vegan Chocolate Orange Truffles
MONDAY	Keto Chicken Salad	Bacon Cheeseburger Soup	Coconut Oil Keto Bombs	Hearty Chicken Stew	Keto Chips with Zucchini
TUESDAY	Tuna, Greens, and Eggs Salad	Creamy Taco Soup (Low Carb)	Keto Easter «Cake»	Beef Stew	Festive Keto Terrine
WEDNESDAY	Tuna, Greens, and Eggs Salad	Wine-Coffee Beef Stew	Buffalo Deviled Eggs	Low Carb Pork Pie	Lemon Cheesecake
THURSDAY	Greek Salad	Keto Creamy Chicken Bacon Soup (instant pot)	Raspberry Lemon Ice Bombs	Green Chile Pork Stew	Keto Livers Truffles
FRIDAY	Keto Cheese Rolls	Stroganoff Soup Keto	Chocolate-Coconut Keto Candies	Venison Spring Keto Stew	Chocolate Keto Ice Cream
SATURDAY	Stuffed Cheese Bell Pepper	Japanese Clear Onion Soup	Keto bombs with Philadelphia Cream Cheese	Low Carb Pork Pie	Chocolate Coconut Fat Bombs

Week 3 Shopping List

PANTRY STAPLES
Butter
Cocoa powder -1 oz.
Coconut Milk – 2 pack
Coconut oil – 10 oz.
Canned tuna -4 can (16 oz.)
Campari tomatoes – 3 lb.

DAIRY & MEAT
Heavy Cream –10 oz.
Soft Cream Cheese –8 containers (48 oz.)
Feta cheese – 8 oz.
Cheddar Cheese – 2 oz.
Eggs – 30 total
Bacon slices –25 oz.
Mascarpone – 5 oz.
Pork tenderloin –5 lb.
Chicken – 24 oz.
Chicken breast – 16 oz.
Chicken liver – 4 oz.
Mozzarella –8 oz.
Beef sirloin 2 lb.
Beef snack, tail -5 lb.
Sour cream – 24 oz.
Ground pork - 1 lb.
Parmesan cheese grated – 10 oz.
Diced tomatoes – 5 oz.
Beef Stew –6 lb.
Venison – 1 lb.

VEGETABLES
Avocados – 2 total
Bell peppers – 12 oz.
Lettuce - 16 oz.
Onions – 7 total
Lemon – 5 total
Cauliflower - ½ lb.
Spinach – 10 oz.
Olives –16 oz.
Zucchini – 4 total

OTHER
Mushrooms –16 oz.
Shrimp –1 lb.
Champignons – 24 oz.
Dark chopped chocolate– 2 oz.

Day 15

Low calories day. Try to limit physical activity today.

Keto Caesar Salad
Keto Paleo Scotch Eggs
Grilled Shrimp and Avocado
Braised Beef and Zucchini
Vegan Chocolate Orange Truffles
Fat - 71g   Carbs - 27g   Protein -100g   Calories -1147

Keto Caesar Salad
```
4 serves | 30 min
```

Ingredients

2/3 lb. chicken breasts

3 oz. bacon

½ lb. Romaine lettuce

2 oz. grated Parmesan cheese

1 tbsp. olive oil

½ cup homemade mayonnaise

1 tbsp. Dijon mustard

½ lemon (juice)

2 tbsp. chopped anchovy filets

1 pressed garlic clove (to taste)

Salt and pepper

Directions

Salad

1. Preheat the oven to 400°F. Grease baking sheet. Place the chicken breasts on sheet.
2. Drizzle olive oil on top of the chicken. Add salt and pepper to breasts.
3. Bake the chicken for 20 minutes, until fully cooked.
4. Fry the bacon until crispy in the frying pan.

5. Shred the lettuce and place on plate.
6. Place sliced chicken on plate, crumble bacon on top.
7. Season the salad with dressing and 30 g grated Parmesan.

Dressing

Mix anchovies' filets, homemade mayonnaise, Dijon mustard, lemon juice, 2 tbsp. grated Parmesan cheese, garlic clove, salt and pepper with immersion blender. Chill in the refrigerator.

Fat – 32g   Carbs – 10g   Protein -36g   Calories -468

Keto Paleo Scotch Eggs

```
6 serves | 40 min
```

Ingredients

6 boiled eggs

1 lb. mince pork, beef, or lamb

2 tsp. herbs to taste

1 tsp. onion flake salt

Salt

Directions

1. Hard boil the eggs.
2. Mix minced meat, herbs and salt.
3. Cover the eggs with the meat completely. You can press the meat.
4. Preheat oven to 350°F.
5. Place the scotch eggs on the baking sheet. Brush them with oil. Sprinkle on onion flakes.
6. Bake the eggs for 15-20 minutes until golden all over.

Fat – 11g   Carbs – 1g   Protein -29g   Calories -219

Grilled Shrimp and Avocado
9 serves | 15 min

Ingredients

1 lb. shrimp (16 shrimp)

½ tsp. salt

1 tsp. black pepper

1 tbsp. onion powder

1 lemon

2 tbsp. coconut aminos

2 tbsp. avocado oil

2 ripe Hass avocados

Directions

1. Peel and clean the shrimp. Place them in a bowl.
2. Add salt, coconut aminos, pepper, onion powder. Add the juice of one half of the lemon. Combine.
3. Heat the grill or frying pan. Add avocado oil. Place shrimp in pan and cook for 3 minutes. Flip the shrimp.
4. Remove the shrimp and cool.
5. Peel and mush avocado with the fork. Add a little salt and lemon juice.
6. Put avocado mixture and the shrimp on the plate

Fat – 9g   Carbs – 4g   Protein -14g   Calories -152

Braised Beef and Zucchini
4 serves | 55 min

Ingredients

2/3 lb. beef

1/3 lb. zucchini

1 onion

2 tbsp. butter

Salt

Pepper

Directions

1. Cut beef and onions into small pieces.
2. Put the butter in a frying pan, and add the beef and onions. Fry until golden brown on high heat.
3. Add a little water, cover and stew for one hour on low heat.
4. Cut the zucchini into slices. Add the vegetables and spices to the beef and stew for 30 minutes.

Fat – 18g   Carbs – 3g   Protein -20g   Calories -256

Vegan Chocolate Orange Truffles

8 serves | 10 min

Ingredients

½ cup pitted dates

1 oz. almond meal

1 tbsp. unsweetened cocoa powder

Extra cocoa powder (for rolling the balls)

1 tbsp. orange juice

Zest of 1 lemon

Directions

1. Place pitted dates, almond meal, cocoa powder, orange juice, and lemon zest in a food processor or a powerful blender. Mix well.
2. Make the mixture into balls using your hands. Make 8 truffles.
3. Roll the candies in cocoa powder to taste.

Fat – 2g   Carbs – 10g   Protein -1g   Calories -52

Day 16

Keto Chicken Salad
Bacon Cheeseburger Soup
Coconut Oil Keto Bombs
Hearty Chicken Stew
Keto Chips with Zucchini
Fat - 109g   Carbs - 30g   Protein -126g   Calories -1573

Keto Chicken Salad
2 serves | 20 min

Ingredients

2/3 lb. chicken breast

3 oz. thin-cut bacon slices

½ lb. avocado

½ oz. mixed leaf greens

4 tbsp. Paleo Ranch Dressing

Duck fat for greasing

Directions

1. Preheat the oven to 400°F.
2. Crisp the chicken breasts. Season with salt and pepper.
3. Grease pan with fat. Place breasts skin side down on the pan. Fry for 5-6 minutes. Flip the chicken and cook 30 seconds. Than transfer pan in the oven. Cook 10-15 minutes, until chicken is cooked through.
4. Place the slices bacon on the bake sheet. Bake the bacon slices in the oven until crispy. Alternatively, crisp the bacon in a frying pan.
5. Remove chicken from the oven. Cool for 5 minutes.
6. Slice the avocado and cooked chicken.
7. Place leafy greens on the plate. Add avocado, crispy bacon and sliced chicken.
8. Top with Ranch dressing.

Fat – 48g   Carbs – 12g   Protein -48g   Calories -627

Bacon Cheeseburger Soup
6 serves | 40 min

Ingredients

5 slices bacon

2/3 lb. ground beef

2 tbsp. butter

3 cups beef broth

½ tsp. garlic powder

½ tsp. onion powder

2 tsp. yellow mustard

½ tsp. black pepper

½ tsp. ground red pepper

1 tsp. cumin

1 tsp. chili powder

2 ½ tbsp. tomato paste

3 medium diced dill pickle

1 cup shredded cheddar cheese

3 oz. cream cheese

½ cup heavy cream

Directions

1. Preheat the frying pan over medium heat. Place strips of bacon in it. Fry bacon for 5 minutes.
2. Remove bacon from the pan. Cook ground beef in the bacon grease for 10-15 minutes.
3. Take the other pan, preheat it. Place butter and spices in it. Cook for 45 seconds.
4. Add broth, mustard, tomato paste, cream cheese to the pan. Cook for 5 minutes, until cream cheese is melting.
5. Add pickles, heavy cream to the sauce, cook until of creamy brown texture.
6. Pour sauce over beef in a frying pan, and add bacon. Simmer for about 5-10 minutes.

Fat – 30g   Carbs – 5g   Protein -32g   Calories -419

Coconut Oil Keto Bombs
10 serves | 10 min

Ingredients

4 oz. cream cheese

1/2 cup heavy cream, whipped

1 tsp. orange vanilla

1/2 cup coconut oil

10 drops of liquid stevia

Directions

1. Mix all ingredients in a blender. Soften them in the microwave if it is difficult to mix the ingredients.
2. Freeze the mixture in silicone molds for 3–4 hours.
3. After freezing, remove the bombs from the molds and store in the refrigerator.

Fat – 19g   Carbs – 1g   Protein -1g   Calories -177

Hearty Chicken Stew
6 serves | 45 min

Ingredients

6 chicken pieces (thighs and legs)

2 small zucchini, sliced into rounds

2 onions

4 medium carrots, peeled and sliced into rounds

2 cups white button mushrooms, halved

2 cups vegetable broth

1 tsp. ground coriander

1 cup baby potatoes

1 tsp. dried thyme

Salt and pepper, to taste

Directions

1. Fry chicken, seasoned with thyme, coriander, salt, and pepper on a heated large pot until the skin has browned.
2. Mix all ingredients in the pot and bring it to a boil. Simmer for about 30 minutes, covered.

Fat – 11g   Carbs – 12g   Protein -44g   Calories -333

Keto Chips with Zucchini

10 serves | 1 h 30 min

Ingredients

1 small zucchini, peeled, chopped

1 oz. sunflower seeds

1/2 tsp. salt, or to taste

1/2 tsp. paprika, or to taste

1/4 tsp. turmeric, or to taste

1/4 tsp. hot pepper flakes, or to taste

Directions

1. Put chopped zucchini and sunflower seeds into a blender.
2. Add spices to the mixture and blend.
3. Preheat the oven to 190°F.
4. Put the mixture on a baking sheet lined with parchment paper. Smooth it out to a thickness of about 1/4 inch.
5. Bake the zucchini mixture for 1–1 1/2 hours. If the chips are non-crunchy after that, bake for a little longer.
6. Remove from the oven and let cool a little before cutting or breaking into 10 chips. (A pizza cutter is ideal for this).

Fat – 1g   Carbs – 1g   Protein -1g   Calories -17

Day 17

Tuna, Greens, and Eggs Salad
Creamy Taco Soup (Low Carb)
Keto Easter «Cake»
Beef Stew
Festive Keto Terrine
Fat - 86g   Carbs - 29g   Protein -137g   Calories -1622

Tuna, Greens, and Eggs Salad
4 serves | 30 min

Ingredients

1/3 lb. canned tuna

¼ lb. lettuce

2 chicken eggs

1 medium onion

2 tbsp. mayonnaise

lemon juice

salt

Directions

1. Cut the lettuce and put it on the plate.
2. Open the can and remove the tuna. Cut pieces, if necessary.
3. Mince the onion, and put it on the fish.
4. Boil the eggs. Cut them in half lengthwise.
5. Season the salad with mayo. Add a couple drops of lemon juice and salt.

Fat – 9g   Carbs – 5g   Protein -15g   Calories -167

Creamy Taco Soup (Low Carb)
6 serves | 1 h 20 min

Ingredients

<u>Soup:</u>

2 tsp. avocado oil (or butter)

1 onion

1 lb. ground beef

2 tbsp. taco seasoning

1 14-oz. cans diced tomatoes

2 cups chicken broth

1/2 cup ranch dressing

1/3 lb. cream cheese

<u>Toppings:</u>

1 oz. sliced olives

3 sliced green onions

2 oz. cilantro fresh (to taste)

1/2 avocado (optional)

1/2 cup cheddar cheese

1/2 cup sour cream

Directions

1. Take a small stock pot. Melt the butter in it over medium heat.
2. Peel and chop the onions, add to the pot. Stir onions occasionally until translucent.
3. Add ground beef and taco seasoning. Cook until ground beef is brown.
4. Add diced tomatoes.
5. Stir in broth, mix well. Simmer for about 20-30 minutes.
6. Add ranch dressing, cream cheese. Cook until cream cheese is melting, for 5 minutes.
7. Add salt and pepper to taste.
8. After cooking, serve soup and garnish with cheddar cheese, chopped green onion, sour cream, cilantro, avocado, and olives.

Fat – 26g   Carbs – 11g   Protein -36g   Calories -575

Keto Easter "Cake"
1 serves | 30 min

Ingredients

9 oz. of soft cream cheese (such as mascarpone)

7 oz. butter at room temperature

1 tsp. sweetener (granulated stevia)

A pinch of vanilla

2 oz. of full-fat sour cream sweetened with 1 tsp. sweetener (for example, stevia)

Directions

1. Mix cream cheese with butter adding sweetener, vanilla extract, and blueberries
2. Completely fill the mold (for the big cupcake) and refrigerate for at least two hours.
3. Turn the mold over and gently remove the "cake".
4. Serve with the sweetened sour cream.

Note: It is not a cottage cheese Easter cake, but it's very, very keto.

Fat – 16g   Carbs – 2g   Protein -3g   Calories -158

Beef Stew
6 serves | 4 h

Ingredients

5 lb. beef snack, tail

3 medium carrots

8 Campari tomatoes

2 medium onions

1 tsp. tomato sauce

8 cloves garlic

2 tsp. garlic powder

2 tbsp. apple cider vinegar

4 cups chicken broth

2 cups water

2 tsp. onion powder

4 tsp. salt

3 tsp. crushed red pepper

2 tsp. parsley

1 tsp. cayenne

2 tsp. black pepper

2 tsp. basil

3 whole bay leaves, spices, to taste

Directions

1. Pell and cut carrots, tomatoes, onion, garlic into chunky pieces.
2. Preheat the frying pan over medium heat.
3. Place vegetables and spices on the frying pan, stir and cook until translucent.
4. Replace the ingredients in the soup pot.
5. Take another cast iron skillet. Place beef snack in it. Cook on both sides, until crispy.
6. Pour broth into the pot to the onion, carrot and garlic.
7. Add two cups of water, apple cider vinegar. Cook for 2-3 minutes. Stir.
8. Add tomatoes, tomato sauce. Stir well.
9. Submerge beef tails into the broth. Boil the ingredients.
10. Reduce the heat to a simmer. Cover the pot.
11. Slightly simmer on a low heat for 3 hours.
12. When meat is cooked, it will be very soft and tender.
13. Remove the bay leaves from the pot. Serve.

Fat – 22g   Carbs – 9g   Protein -68g   Calories -531

Festive Keto Terrine
8 serves | 1 hour (+ 10 hours in the fridge)

Ingredients

5 oz. Mascarpone cheese

2 oz. full-fat sour cream

1 lb. skin-less, bone-less chicken breast fillets

5 oz. heavy cream

2 tsp. gelatin

3 tbsp. hot water

1/2 tsp. salt and pepper or to taste

1/2 tbsp. black sesame seeds

Greens of your choice for serving

Directions

1. Cut chicken breast into cubes and boil them for 15 minutes.
2. Dissolve gelatin completely in the hot water and let it swell. Pour it into the sour cream.
3. Add salt and pepper to taste to the sour cream and gelatin.
4. Pour the mixture into a terrine mold. Place the mold in the fridge.
5. While the sour cream is cooling, whip the heavy cream with mascarpone cheese for about 1–2 minutes. Add salt and pepper.

6. Add chilled pieces of chicken and sesame seeds, and mix well.
7. When the gelatin-sour cream mixture has set, spoon the chicken mixture on top.
8. Place the dish in the fridge overnight.
9. In the morning remove the terrine from the mold by inverting it over a plate. If the mixture is stuck in the mold. Warm it slightly in warm water or with a hair dryer and run a knife around the side. Do not make it too warm.
10. Use a second plate and invert the terrine once more so the bottom of the terrine is now on the plate.
11. Sprinkle the terrine with finely chopped greens, cranberries or some other garnish of your choice.

Fat – 13g   Carbs – 2g   Protein -15g   Calories -192

Day 18

Tuna, Greens, and Eggs Salad
Wine-Coffee Beef Stew
Buffalo Deviled Eggs
Low Carb Pork Pie
Lemon Cheesecake
Fat - 92g   Carbs - 17g   Protein -128g   Calories -1410

Tuna, Greens, and Eggs Salad

4 serves | 30 min

Ingredients

1/3 lb. canned tuna

¼ lb. lettuce

2 eggs

1 medium onion

2 tbsp. mayonnaise

Lemon juice

Salt

Directions

1. Cut the lettuce and put it on the plate.
2. Open the can and remove the tuna. Cut pieces, if necessary.
3. Mince the onion, and put it on the fish.
4. Boil the eggs. Cut them in half lengthwise.
5. Season the salad with mayo. Add a couple drops of lemon juice and salt.

Fat – 9g   Carbs – 5g   Protein -15g   Calories -167

Wine-Coffee Beef Stew

6 serves | 3 h 30 min

Ingredients

- 3 lb. stew meat
- 3 cups coffee
- 1 cup beef stock
- 1 ½ cup baby bella mushrooms
- 2/3 cup red wine
- 1 medium onion
- 3 tbsp. coconut oil
- 2 tbsp. capers
- 2 tsp. garlic
- 1 tsp. salt
- 1 tsp. pepper

Directions

1. Cut all stew meat in cubes.
2. Slice onions and mushrooms thinly.
3. Take a deep frying pan; pour 3 tbsp. coconut oil in it. Preheat the frying pan.
4. Place beef on the pan. Season beef with salt and pepper.
5. Fry meat in small batches. Place all meat in the pan after browning.
6. Place onion, mushrooms in the saucepan with the remaining fat. Cook until onion is translucent.
7. Pour coffee, beef stock, red wine, add capers to the vegetables and stir this mixture.
8. Add beef into the mixture, bring to a boil, and then reduce the heat to low.
9. Cover and cook for 3 hours.

Fat – 32g   Carbs – 3g   Protein -43g   Calories -504

Buffalo Deviled Eggs

6 serves | 30 min

Ingredients

6 hard boiled chicken eggs, large

1/3 lb. boiled and chopped chicken

¼ onion

¼ cup blue cheese crumbles

¼ cup Franks Buffalo Wing Sauce

1 small chopped celery

2 tbsp. blue cheese dressing

Directions

1. Boil the eggs.
2. Chop the chicken and celery.
3. Peel cooked and cooled eggs. Cut them in half lengthwise. Separate the yolks from the egg whites and place yolks in mixing bowl.
4. Add chicken, celery, blue cheese, Franks Buffalo Wing Sauce and dressing to yolks.
5. Press the onion and add juice to the bowl. Mix all the ingredients.
6. Stuff the egg whites with yolk mixture using a fork or spoon. You can also pipe the yolks into the whites using a Ziploc bag with the tip cut off.

Fat – 12g   Carbs – 2g   Protein -29g   Calories -152

Low Carb Pork Pie
4 serves | 1 h 15 min

Ingredients

1 lb. ground pork

4 tbsp. grated Parmesan cheese

2 large eggs

½ lemon zest

½ tsp. ground nutmeg

½ tsp. ginger

½ tsp. cardamom

4 tart shells

Salt and pepper to taste

Directions

1. Heat a pan. Add meat and spices. Cook for 10-15 minutes over medium heat, and then remove a pan from heat. Add the eggs, cheese, and lemon zest.
2. Preheat the oven to 325 °F.
3. Place mixture into pie shells. Bake for 20-25 minutes in oven.
4. Remove pie from the oven. Let cool and serve.

Fat – 12g   Carbs – 5g   Protein -36g   Calories -317

Lemon Cheesecake
4 serves | 10 min

Ingredients

½ lb. soft cream cheese

2 oz. fatty cream

1 tbsp. lemon juice

1 tsp. stevia in liquid form

1 tsp. lemon peel

vanilla

Directions

1. Put cream cheese and cream on a bowl. Mix them with a mixer until uniform mass.
2. Add stevia, lemon juice, vanilla, lemon zest. Mix well.
3. Put the mixture into tart pans you may consume immediately. For best results, chill in the refrigerator for two hours to harden.

Fat – 27g   Carbs – 3g   Protein -6g   Calories -270

Day 19

Low calories day. Try to limit physical activity today.

Greek Salad
Keto Creamy Chicken Bacon Soup (instant pot)
Raspberry Lemon Ice Bombs
Green Chile Pork Stew
Keto Livers Truffles
Fat - 132g   Carbs – 31g   Protein -121g   Calories -1152

Greek Salad
4 serves | 15 min

Ingredients

2 ripe tomatoes

½ cucumber

½ red onion

½ green bell pepper

½ lb. Feta cheese

10 black olives

2 tbsp. olive oil

½ tbsp. red wine vinegar

2 tsp. dried oregano

Salt and pepper

Directions

Salad

1. Cut the tomatoes and cucumber into bite-sized pieces.
2. Thinly slice the bell pepper and onion.
3. Arrange the ingredients on a plate.
4. Add feta and olives.
5. Drizzle the salad with the dressing.
6. Sprinkle with oregano.

Dressing

Mix the olive oil and vinegar. Add salt and pepper to taste.

Fat – 20g   Carbs – 10g   Protein -9g   Calories -252

Creamy Chicken Bacon Soup (instant pot)

6 serves | 40 min

Ingredients

6 chicken thighs, boneless

½ lb. cream cheese full fat

3 tsp. minced garlic

1 cup frozen the chopped onion-celery mix

1/3 lb. sliced mushrooms

4 tsp. butter

1 tsp. thyme

Salt and pepper to taste

3 cups chicken broth

1 cup heavy cream

1 lb. chopped cooked bacon

2 cups fresh spinach

Directions

1. Cut chicken thighs into cubes, place into a large zipper bag.
2. Add full-fat cream cheese, minced garlic, frozen chopped onion-celery mix, sliced mushrooms, butter, thyme, salt, and pepper to taste to the zipper bag. Place the bag in a fridge.
3. At the same time pour chicken mixture into Instant Pot.
4. Add chicken broth and cook for 30 minutes. Use the soup setting.
5. Mix well the ingredients, add spinach and cream.
6. Cover the instant pot and let it sit for 10 minutes until spinach wilt.
7. At the same time slice and cut the bacon. Place the slices in the frying pan. Cook for 5 minutes.
8. Pour the soup in a bowl and top with fried bacon.

Fat – 63g   Carbs – 7g   Protein -77g   Calories -452

Raspberry Lemon Ice Bombs
6 serves | 2 h 30 min

Ingredients

1/4 cup coconut oil

1 cup coconut milk

1/4 cup sour cream

1/4 cup cream

3 1/2 oz. raspberries

Juice of half a lemon

20 drops liquid stevia

Directions

1. Put all the ingredients in a blender and blend until the raspberries mix with the rest of the products.
2. Strain the mixture to remove the raspberry seeds. It's important because the seeds in the finished ice bombs will irritate the tongue.
3. Pour the mixture into 5 silicone molds and freeze for two hours.

Fat – 25g   Carbs – 6g   Protein -2g   Calories -246

Green Chile Pork Stew

8 serves | 1 h 45 min

Ingredients

2 lb. pork loin

2 tsp. ground cumin

2 tsp. granulated garlic

1 tsp. pure ground Chile powder (to taste)

2 oz. chopped onion

Two cloves garlic

3 cups whole hatch green chilies and liquid

3 tbsp. oil

2 cups water

Poached eggs optional

Salt to taste

Directions

1. Cut pork loin into cubes.
2. Preheat oil in a big frying pan. Fry pork until brown.
3. Add spices to the pork. Cook until fragrant.
4. At the same time chop garlic and onion. Place ingredients in a food processor.
5. Add canned chilies to the food processor. Mix and make thick chunky paste.

6. Add chili and onion mixture to the pork. Pour the liquid of canned chilies.

7. Pour two cups of water.

8. Stir the ingredients and make low-heat. Cover the pan with a lid.

9. Simmer the stew for 60-90 minutes until pork is tender.

10. Add a little water during the last hour cooking.

11. Before finishing, add salt to taste.

12. Serve stew with the poached eggs.

Fat – 10g   Carbs – 4g   Protein -20g   Calories -182

Keto Livers Truffles

12 serves | 50 min

Ingredients

3 oz. soft cheese

7 oz. chicken livers

1 tsp. butter

1 tbsp. cognac

1–2 tbsp. cocoa powder

1–2 tbsp. mixture of seeds (chia, sesame, flax seed)

olive oil, salt, pepper

Directions

1. Preheat a frying pan. Cook the livers in olive oil for 5 minutes on high heat. Add cognac and flame it or you can just let it evaporate. Reduce the heat, add the butter and continue cooking the livers until done. Remove the livers from the pan and allow them to cool.
2. Mix cold livers with the cheese in a food processor. Put liver-cheese mix in the fridge before forming truffles.
3. Make 12 balls from liver-cheese mixture (wet hands will be better). Roll some balls into the cocoa and some into the mixture of seeds. Serve.

Note: If you are having a buffet, serve the truffles in a small paper basket as for homemade chocolates.

Fat – 2g   Carbs – 1g   Protein -5g   Calories -40

Day 20

Keto Cheese Rolls
Stroganoff Soup Keto
Chocolate-Coconut Keto Candies
Venison Spring Keto Stew
Chocolate Keto Ice Cream
Fat - 100g   Carbs - 31g   Protein -98g   Calories -1420

Keto Cheese Rolls

3 serves | 30 min

Ingredients

4 eggs, separated

1 clove of garlic, peeled and crushed

2 oz. hard cheese, grated

4 tbsp. homemade mayonnaise

3 oz. cauliflower (can be frozen), blanched

2 pieces of melted cheese

black pepper to taste

1 bunch greens to taste, chop finely

Directions

1. Grind blanched cauliflower in a blender or grinder for 5 minutes.
2. Beat egg whites into a creamy foam and set aside.
3. Preheat oven to 350°F.
4. Line a baking sheet with parchment paper.
5. Mix cauliflower with yolks, and then gently fold in the whites.
6. Put the mixture on the baking sheet and smooth it out. Place it in the oven for 15 minutes.
7. Mix the grated cheese with garlic, spices, salt, greens and homemade mayonnaise for the toppings.
8. After baking, remove the base from the oven. Place the toppings on it and spread it over the base. Take one edge of the base and gently roll it like a jelly-roll. Lay it on a plate and slice the roll into 3 portions.

Fat – 20g   Carbs – 9g   Protein -15g   Calories -269

Stroganoff High Fat Soup
6 serves | 1 h

Ingredients

2 lb. sirloin beef

1 ½ lb. champignon

2 oz. ghee

2 cloves minced garlic

¼ lb. medium chopped white onion

5 cups bone, chicken or vegetable broth

2 tsp. paprika

1 tbsp. Dijon mustard

4 tbsp. lemon juice

2/3 lb. sour cream

1/4 cup freshly chopped parsley

1 tsp. salt

1/4 tsp. freshly ground black pepper

Directions

1. Slice beef into thin strips. Season with some salt and pepper.
2. Clean and slice the mushrooms.
3. Grease a large, heavy bottom pan with half of the ghee. Preheat the pan. Try to add beef in one layer. Fry slices over

medium-high heat quickly until the meat becomes brown on all sides. Repeat for the remaining slices.

4. Remove slices from the pan, place them in a bowl. Set aside.

5. Grease a pan with the remaining ghee. Place chopped onion and minced garlic in the pan. Cook for about 2-3 minutes.

6. Add sliced mushrooms to the pan. Cook for 3-5 minutes.

7. Add Dijon mustard, paprika. Mix the ingredients. Pour bone broth in a pan.

8. Add lemon juice and bring to a boil. Cook for 2-3 minutes.

9. Add the browned beef slices and sour cream. Cook for 1-2 minutes, take off the heat.

Fat – 31g   Carbs – 7g   Protein -47g   Calories -520

Chocolate-Coconut Keto Candies
20 serves | 1 h 5 min

Ingredients

2 oz. butter, melted

2 tbsp. coconut flakes

1/2 oz. of any nuts, crushed

1/2 tbsp. cocoa powder

1 tsp. granulated sweetener to taste

1 tsp. vanilla extract

Directions

1. Melt the butter. Mix all ingredients and add them to the melted butter. Stir well.

2. Use a small rectangular mold. Pour the mixture into it. Put the mold into the refrigerator for 1–4 hours.

3. When it is hard, remove it from the refrigerator and cut the hard mass into 20 pieces of candy.

Note: should keep refrigerated.

Fat – 6g   Carbs – 1g   Protein -0g   Calories -54

Venison Spring HFLC Stew
4 serves | 4 h 20 min

Ingredients

1 lb. venison

2 tbsp. olive oil

1 bulb garlic

1 cup shredded cabbage (purple)

1 cup sliced celery

4 cups bone broth

1 tsp. salt

1 tsp. pepper

2 cups chopped asparagus

2 bay leaves

Directions

1. At first, peel and slice garlic. Cut it into 1/8-inch thin slices.
2. Slice the purple cabbage.
3. Slice celery.
4. Preheat the skillet. Pour olive oil in it.
5. Add celery, garlic, bay leaves to the skillet. Saute the ingredients for about 5-6 minutes until tender.
6. Add venison to the cabbage. Salt and pepper. Cook until the meat is brown.
7. Take a big saucepan. Place cabbage and venison in it, add broth.
8. Stew for 4 hours. Add water if the stew is dry.
9. When done, add chopped asparagus in the saucepan.
10. Serve the stew with olive oil and lime.

Fat – 16g   Carbs – 8g   Protein -32g   Calories -310

Chocolate Keto Ice Cream
6 serves | 3 h 20 min

Ingredients

2 1/2 oz. coconut cream

2 oz. butter or coconut oil

1 tbsp. cocoa

1 tsp. vanilla extract

1 2/3 cups coconut milk

1–2 tsp. liquid sweetener

4 egg yolks

1/8 tsp. xanthan gum (optional)

Directions

1. Whisk the egg yolks.
2. On low heat warm 1/2 cup of coconut milk with the vanilla extract in a small saucepan.
3. Stir vanilla milk and pour it slowly in a thin stream into the yolks, stirring gently. Do this gradually so that the eggs yolks do not coagulate. Cook the yolk mixture on low heat, stirring, for 5–7 minutes until the mix thickens. Don't let it boil. After that, cool the mixture down.
4. If you use xanthan gum, mix it with the liquid sweetener.
5. Slowly pour the sweetener into the beaten cold milk mixture, stirring. If you prefer not to use the xanthan gum, you can pour all the sweetener at once into the milk.
6. 6. Then gently mix the coconut milk-yolk mixture with the cocoa, butter or oil, and the coconut cream. Beat all ingredients together for 1–2 minutes.

7. You can use an ice cream maker for freezing the mixture.
8. Put the ice cream into the freezer for about 3–4 hours.

Note: This keto ice cream is for those who do not eat dairy products but, at the same time, love ice cream.

Fat – 27g   Carbs – 6g   Protein -3g   Calories -267

Day 21

Low calories day. Try to limit physical activity today.

Stuffed Cheese Bell Pepper
Japanese Clear Onion Soup
Keto bombs with Philadelphia Cream Cheese
Low Carb Pork Pie
Chocolate Coconut Fat Bombs
Fat - 46g   Carbs - 31g   Protein -55g   Calories -1091

Stuffed Cheese Bell Pepper

4 serves | 45 min

Ingredients

2 bell peppers, 2/3 lb.

2 chicken eggs

4 oz. mozzarella cheese

4 oz. Parmesan cheese

4 oz. ricotta cheese

3 tbsp. dried parsley

1 cup spinach

salt

Directions

1. Preheat the oven to 370ºF.
2. Wash and peel the peppers. Cut them in half lengthwise.
3. Mix cheese, eggs, and dried parsley in a blender.
4. Stuff each half with cheese mixture.
5. Put spinach on the top of the pepper. Bake for 30 min.
6. Sprinkle the Parmesan on the peppers and return to the oven for 5 min.

Fat – 9g   Carbs – 10g   Protein -15g   Calories -169

Japanese Clear Onion Soup

4 serves | 40 min

Ingredients

2 onions, diced

6 cups water or vegetable broth

2 celery stalks, diced

2 carrots, diced

2 cloves of garlic

2 oz. button mushrooms, sliced

2 oz. scallions

1 tbsp. olive oil

salt, pepper, soy sauce, Sriracha sauce, to taste

Directions

1. Preheat the oil in a saucepan. Place onions in it. Saute the onions until slightly brown.
2. Add peeled and chopped carrots, onions, celery, garlic.
3. Pour 6 cups of water or broth.
4. Boil for 30 minutes.
5. Strain vegetables from the broth.
6. Peel and slice the mushrooms.
7. Cut scallions.
8. Add mushrooms, scallions to the broth before serving.
9. Add soy sauce, Sriracha to taste

Fat – 4g   Carbs – 10g   Protein -2g   Calories -100

Keto bombs with Philadelphia Cream Cheese
8 serves | 40 min

Ingredients

For the bombs:

5 1/2 oz. Philadelphia Cream Cheese

2 oz. butter

2 oz. coconut oil

1/2 tsp. erythritol

To taste granulated or liquid stevia sweetener

Vanilla extract or vanilla pods

For keto chocolate topping:

1 oz. cocoa powder

1 tbsp. coconut oil or cocoa butter

Stevia extract

Directions

1. Mix all the ingredients for the bombs together in a food processor until there is a uniform mixture.
2. Add the erythritol gradually, tasting from time to time for sweetness to your taste. You will need about 1/2 tsp. of erythritol and one drop of stevia. Stir until it is completely dissolved.
3. Using small silicone or muffin molds, transfer the mixture to the molds. Fill them 3/4 full.
4. Place the bombs into the freezer for 15–20 minutes.

5. Meanwhile, prepare the keto chocolate topping. Heat grated cocoa with coconut oil in a water bath. Add only stevia extract for sweetness! Stir. When the mixture becomes well combined, remove from the heat and let cool slightly.
6. Remove the keto bombs from the freezer and pour chocolate mixture on them. Refrigerate for 2 more hours.

Fat – 2g   Carbs – 3g   Protein -1g   Calories -318

Low Carb Pork Pie

4 serves | 1 h 15 min

Ingredients

1 lb. ground pork

4 tbsp. grated Parmesan cheese

2 large eggs

½ lemon zest

½ tsp. ground nutmeg

½ tsp. ginger

½ tsp. cardamom

4 tart shells

salt and pepper to taste

Directions

1. Heat a pan. Add meat and spices. Cook for 10-15 minutes over medium heat, and then remove a pan from heat. Add the eggs, cheese, and lemon zest.
2. Preheat the oven to 325 °F.
3. Place mixture into pie shells. Bake for 20-25 minutes in oven.
4. Remove pie from the oven. Let cool and serve.

Fat – 12g   Carbs – 5g   Protein -36g   Calories -317

Chocolate Coconut Fat Bombs
8 serves | 12 min

Ingredients

1/4 cup savory coconut flakes

1/4 cup liquid coconut oil

2 tbsp. erythritol

1/4 cup solid coconut oil

1 oz. dark chocolate (sugar-free, 85% or more cocoa content)

Directions

1. Melt the mixture of coconut oils in the microwave for 45 seconds to 1 minute and mix well.
2. Add coconut flakes and sweetener, and mix well again.
3. Pour the mixture into ice trays (or silicon molds) and freeze for 30 minutes.
4. Melt dark chocolate in the microwave for 1 minute.
5. Pour equally over each coconut bomb by the spoonful's of chocolate.

Fat – 19g   Carbs – 3g   Protein -1g   Calories -187

Thank you for spending three weeks with us.

We hope that it was tasty, and you have a new habit of high fat low carb eating.

Leave your feedback and suggestions, because we want to become better with you.

Dan Barnett

Mass and Volume Conversion Rates

Imperial		Metric
1 ounce [oz]	437.5 grain	28.35 g
1 pound [lb]	16 oz.	453.6 g
1 cup	8 fl oz	237 ml
1 tbsp.		15 ml
1 tsp.		5 ml

Metric	Imperial	
100 gram [g]	3.52 ounce [oz]	
500 gram [g]	1.1 pound [lb]	
5 ml	1 tsp	1/3 tbsp.
1 liter [l]	4.2 cup	33.2 fl oz

High Fat Low Carb Food List

All values are approximate from Google data, sorted from lowest to highest net carb count.

MEATS

ITEM / WEIGHT	NET CARBS
Bacon (1 Pan fried slice, 10g)	0
Beef (70/30 Ground, 100g)	0
Beef (85/15 Ground, 100g)	0
Beef (Brisket, 100g)	0
Chicken (Breast, 100g)	0
Chicken (Thighs, 100g)	0
Chicken (Drumsticks, 100g)	0
Chicken (Wings, 100g)	0
Crab (King, 100g)	0
Fish (Tuna, 100g)	0
Fish (Tilapia, 100g)	0
Fish (Salmon, 100g)	0
Fish (Catfish, 100g)	0
Fish (Halibut, 100g)	0
Fish (Sole, 85g)	0
Fish (Pacific Cod, 100g)	0
Fish (Pompano, 100g)	0
Lobster (cooked, 100g)	0
Pork (varies, 100g)	0
Turkey (Breast, 100g)	0
Turkey (Leg, 100g)	0
Turkey (Dark Meat, 100g)	0
Shrimp (85g)	0.2
Egg (Large, 50g)	0.4
Chicken (Liver, 100g)	0.7
Scallops (steamed, 100g)	5

HERBS & SPICES

ITEM / WEIGHT	NET CARBS
Cilantro (20g)	0.1
Thyme (0.8g)	0.1
Dill (1g)	0.1
Oregano (2g, ground, dried)	0.2

VEGETABLES

ITEM / WEIGHT	NET CARBS
Collard Greens (100g)	1
Lettuce (Romaine, 100g)	1.2
Bok Choy (100g)	1.2
Spinach (100g)	1.4
Lettuce (Green Leaf, 100g)	1.6
Celery (100g)	1.7
Asparagus (100g)	1.8
Radishes (100g)	1.8
Avocado (100g)	2
Cabbage (Napa, 100g)	2
Arugula (100g)	2.1
Mushrooms (White, 100g)	2.3
Yellow Squash (100g)	2.3
Zucchini (100g)	2.4
Mushrooms (Portobello, 100g)	2.6
Tomato (Red, 100g)	2.7
Olives (100g)	2.8
Bell Pepper (Green, 100g)	2.9
Eggplant (100g)	3
Cauliflower (100g)	3
Cucumbers (100g)	3.1
Cabbage (Green, 100g)	3.5
Green Beans (100g)	3.6
Bell Pepper (Red, 100g)	3.9
Kale (Boiled, 100g)	4
Jalapeno (100g)	4.2
Broccoli (100g)	4.4
Green Onions (100g)	4.4
Cabbage (Red, 100g)	4.7
Edamame (100g)	5
Bell Pepper (Yellow, 100g)	5.3
Brussel Sprouts (100g)	5.2
Spaghetti Squash (100g)	5.5
Artichokes (100g)	6

DAIRY

ITEM / WEIGHT	NET CARBS
Pepper Jack (28g / 1oz)	0
Monterey Jack (28g / 1oz)	0
Butter (1 tbsp)	0
Butter, Whipped (1 tbsp)	0
Cheddar (28g / 1oz)	0.4
Heavy Cream (1 tbsp)	0.4
Mozzarella (28g / 1oz, Whole Milk)	0.5
Blue Cheese (28g / 1oz)	0.7
Mozzarella (28g / 1oz, Skim Milk)	0.8
Half & Half (2 tbsp)	1
Parmesan (28g / 1oz)	1.2
Feta (28g / 1oz)	1.2
Cream Cheese (28g / 1oz)	1.2
Swiss (28g / 1oz)	1.5
Ricotta Cheese (100g)	3
Cottage Cheese (100g)	3.4

NOTES

171

Printed in Great Britain
by Amazon